HARDCORE Microbiology and Immunology

HARDCORE Microbiology and Immunology

Benjamin W. Sears, MD
Orthopedic Surgery Resident
Loyola University Medical Center
Chicago, Illinois

Lisa M. Spear, MD
Emergency Medicine Resident
University of Illinois at Chicago Medical Center
Chicago, Illinois

Rodrigo Saenz, MD
Radiology Resident
University of South Florida Health Sciences Center
Tampa, Florida

Original art by Kimberly Battista

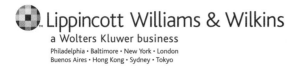. Lippincott Williams & Wilkins
a Wolters Kluwer business
Philadelphia · Baltimore · New York · London
Buenos Aires · Hong Kong · Sydney · Tokyo

Acquisitions Editor: Nancy Anastasi Duffy
Developmental Editor: Kathleen H. Scogna
Production Editor: Kevin P. Johnson
Marketing Manager: Emilie Linkins
Compositor: International Typesetting and Composition

351 West Camden Street
Baltimore, MD 21201

530 Walnut Street
Philadelphia, PA 19106

Printed in the United States of America

First Edition, 1996

Library of Congress Cataloging-in-Publication Data

Sears, Benjamin W.
   Hardcore microbiology and immunology / Benjamin Sears, Lisa M. Spear, Rodrigo Saenz ; original art by Kimberly Battista.
       p. ; cm.—(Hardcore series)
   Includes index.
     ISBN-13: 978-1-4051-0486-9
     ISBN-10: 1-4051-0486-4
     1. Medical microbiology—Examinations, questions, etc. 2. Medical immunology—Examinations, questions, etc. 3. Communicable diseases—Examinations, questions, etc. I. Spear, Lisa M. II. Saenz, Rodrigo E. III. Title. IV. Series.
       [DNLM: 1. Communicable Diseases—microbiology—Examination Questions. 2. Communicable Diseases—microbiology—Outlines. 3. Immune System—Examination Questions. 4. Immune System—Outlines. 5. Immune System Diseases—Examination Questions. 6. Immune System Diseases—Outlines.   WC 18.2 S439h 2006]
   QR46.S43 2006
   616.9'041—dc22

2006015065

To purchase additional copies of this book, call our customer service department at **(800) 638-3030** or fax orders to **(301) 223-2320.** International customers should call **(301) 223-2300.**

Visit Lippincott Williams & Wilkins on the Internet: http://www.LWW.com. Lippincott Williams & Wilkins customer service representatives are available from 8:30 am to 6:00 pm, EST.

06 07 08 09 10
1 2 3 4 5 6 7 8 9 10

This book is dedicated to our parents and families for their unconditional support and encouragement during the last four years of medical school.

This book is also dedicated to Jim Verseman, whose zest for living and unwavering positive outlook on life should be an inspiration to us all.

About the Authors

Benjamin W. Sears, MD

Ben Sears was born in Fort Collins, Colorado in 1977. He grew up in Aurora, Colorado before attending Colorado State University in Fort Collins. In 2000, he graduated from CSU with a Bachelor of Science in Zoology and a Minor in Nutrition. In 2001, he earned a Master of Science degree in Pharmacology from Tulane University in New Orleans, Louisiana. In 2005, Ben received his Medical Doctorate degree from the Loyola Stritch School of Medicine in Chicago and began his residency at Loyola in Orthopaedic Surgery.

Lisa M. Spear, MD

Lisa Spear was born and raised in Sacramento, California. She completed her Bachelor of Science degree in Exercise Sports Science at Pepperdine University in Malibu, California in 1998. Lisa spent the next three years serving celebrities cocktails in Malibu and conducting research for the University of California at Los Angeles Department of Geriatrics. In 2005, Lisa earned her Medical Doctorate degree from the Loyola Stritch School of Medicine in Chicago. She is currently in her residency in the Department of Emergency Medicine at the University of Illinois Medical Center in Chicago, Illinois.

Rodrigo Saenz, MD

Rodrigo Saenz was born in Panama City, Panama. He completed college with a Bachelor of Science degree in Biology from the University of Louisiana at Lafayette in 1998 and a Master of Science in Pharmacology from Tulane University in 2001. Rodrigo received his Medical Doctorate degree in May 2005 from the Louisiana State University Health Sciences Center School of Medicine in New Orleans and will complete his internship from LSU Medical Center in June 2006 and begin his Radiology residency at Southern Florida University Medical Center in Tampa, Florida.

A Note to the Reader

The Hardcore Board Review series was created during the end of our second year of medical school while preparing for the USMLE Step 1 examination. During this important but difficult time, we realized that, despite the library of Step 1 "review texts" there was actually a void in useful review material for most subjects which provided fast and effective review. Although many available texts are helpful for learning new material and preparing for medical school exams, these same texts are overloaded with unnecessary detail and are cumbersome to navigate during the limited time a student has to review for the board exam. We have designed our Hardcore series to provide you with only the essential information tested on the USMLE Step 1, and presented in a concise, well-organized, and simple format that can be completely reviewed in a short amount of time.

Microbiology comprises a substantial component of the Step 1 exam (approximately 20–40%). Given the breadth and diversity of the material, reviewing it can be both daunting and frustrating. While sifting through numerous "sources" of review material and attempting countless board-style questions while studying for the exam, we were happy to discover that an increasing percentage of microbiology questions were actually clinical in nature. We discovered that many of the infectious diseases tested on Step 1 could be categorized based on the clinical scenario presented in the question, so we roughly organized these organisms and infectious diseases into categories based on the patient group that was commonly affected by them. After taking the actual board exam, we realized how beneficial this grouping system was, as almost all clinical microbiology questions included a specific demographic in their question stem.

Although the USMLE examination commonly uses test questions that are clinically based, we are aware that basic microbiology concepts and principles are also tested. These concepts must be mastered and often are an important component of test questions, many of which also include a clinical scenario. In this review text, we provide you with a concise but targeted chapter outlining the basics of microbiology that Step 1 will test, as well as a chapter that covers other key concepts, laboratory techniques, common organisms by site of infection, and clinical comparisons. In addition, we realize that a number of organisms may be associated with several different demographic groups. We believe it is imperative to this text to include an appendix that provides a comprehensive source of information for each organism, including microbial key features, virulence and toxins, and all clinical correlations and hardcore microbiology reference points. For such information please refer to Appendix B, Complete Microbial Profile, available at http://connection.lww.com/hardcoremicro.

Although immunology is not as heavily tested on Step 1 as microbiology, immunology concepts are becoming increasingly important clinically and are showing up more frequently on the USMLE exam. These concepts are obviously linked closely with microbiology and we believe it is most effective to study these concepts together. Immunology is a challenging subject to master, so we have simply included the components of the immune system (the players), the functions of the immune system (the game), and clinical correlations that you may be tested on. We believe this is the most effective and focused way to review this material.

This book is designed by students who recently took the USMLE Step 1, for students with limited time to review the concepts of medical microbiology and immunology for this increasingly important exam. We believe this is one of the most hardcore, high-yield, yet comprehensive review books available, and we hope that you find this text as useful as we believe it would have been to us while preparing to take Step 1.

Reviewers

Suzanne Bentley
MS 3, University of Medicine and Dentistry of New Jersey
Newark, New Jersey

Alexandra Binnie
MS 3, Harvard University Medical School
Boston, Massachusetts

Rachael Chambers
Resident, Duluth Family Practice Residency Program
Duluth, Minnesota

Olga Fedin
MS 3, UCLA David Geffen School of Medicine
Los Angeles, California

Roxanne Landesman
MS 3, Harvard University Medical School
Boston, Massachusetts

David Lawrence
MS 2, Drexel University College of Medicine
Philadelphia, Pennsylvania

Linda McMurphy
MS 3, University of Oklahoma College of Medicine
Oklahoma City, Oklahoma

Nicolas Pfleghaar
MS 1, Medical University of Ohio
Toledo, Ohio

Daniel Saddawi-Konefka
MS 2, University of Michigan Medical School
Ann Arbor, Michigan

T. Renee Williams
MS 3, Meharry Medical College School of Medicine
Nashville, Tennessee

Anthony Wang
MS 3, Duke University School of Medicine
Durham, North Carolina

Acknowledgments

This book would have never have been possible without the contributions and criticism of the following very important people.

We would like to thank Dr. David Daniels, Internal Medicine Resident, Stanford University, for contributing to the concept of a demographic-based microbiology text for medical students preparing for Step1.

Thanks to Dr. Gadiel Bersrio for his contribution to this text, particularly with the concepts presented in the immunology chapters.

Thanks to Dr. Rolando Saenz, Professor of Medicine, School of Medicine, University Medical Center, Lafayette, Louisiana for his critique and review of this manuscript.

Thanks to Bill Wilson, long-time friend and journalist from Longmont, Colorado, for his support of this text. Sorry about the spill, but you knew what was coming.

Thanks to Caribou Coffee in Oak Park, Illinois for keeping us focused and happy.

Thanks to Beverly Copland, formerly of Blackwell Publishing, for giving us the chance to create the Hardcore series, as well as for pushing us to create and develop Hardcore Microbiology and Immunology, which would have never happened without her unquestioned support and stubbornness.

And, a considerable amount of thanks to Lippincott Williams & Wilkins for their support and publication of this project, in particular Kathleen Scogna, Senior Developmental Editor, artist Kim Battista, and Nancy Duffy, Acquisitions Editor. Their insight and ideas have been crucial to the development and completion of this text.

Contents

CHAPTER 1

Hardcore Introduction to Microbiology

The basic principles of medical microbiology outlined in this chapter are fundamental to understanding the concepts tested on Step 1. On your test, you will be asked to identify organisms based on their structural components or laboratory properties. You will need to understand the differences between gram-positive and gram-negative bacteria, which viruses are RNA viruses and which are DNA viruses, and which properties allow microorganisms to invade the human host and cause disease. This chapter provides you with an explanation of these concepts, which are heavily tested on Step 1, as well as an overview of many organisms that are discussed in further detail throughout the book.

I. BACTERIA

A. Cell Walls and the Gram Stain

Gram stain is a staining process that uses a **crystal violet stain** (which is *blue*) and a **safranin stain** (which is *red*) to separate bacteria into two categories based on properties of the organism's cell wall (Fig. 1-1). This laboratory procedure begins by coating specimens with the blue-appearing crystal violet stain. Next, the organisms are thoroughly rinsed and the red-staining safranin stain is applied. Based on the properties of their cell walls, certain organisms absorb the crystal violet stain into the cell wall and maintain it during rinsing, ultimately *staining blue; these organisms are called* **gram-positive**. Organisms that do not retain the crystal violet stain during rinsing will stain red with the subsequent safranin stain and *appear red; these organisms are called* **gram-negative**.

- *Gram-positive organisms* have a thick outer cell wall made of complex polymers called **peptidoglycans**. Gram-negative organisms also possess a peptidoglycan layer, but it is much thinner. In addition, the gram-positive cell walls contain many cross-linked amino-acid side chains that create a complex layer resembling a barbed-wire fence. When the crystal violet stain is

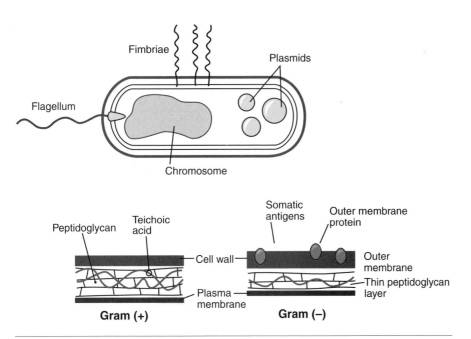

Figure 1–1 Overview of bacterial structure. Important structures include the cell capsule, which protects the organism from phagocytosis and desiccation; lipopolysaccharide, which protects gram-negative bacteria from complement lysis and stimulates cytokines; fimbriae, which helps the cell adhere to host cells; and flagella, which assist in locomotion.

applied, the dye becomes trapped in the complex "barbed" cell wall of gram-positive organisms, staining *blue*.

- In contrast, the thin *gram-negative organisms* are unable to trap the crystal violet stain. The stain is easily rinsed off the simple gram-negative cell wall, allowing the safranin to stain these organisms *red*.

- Another important difference between gram-positive and gram-negative organisms' cell structures is the unique *outer cell membrane of gram-negative organisms*. Whereas the outermost layer of gram-positive organisms is the thick, cross-linked peptidoglycan cell wall, gram-negative organisms have an outer phospholipid bilayer containing **lipopolysaccharide (LPS)**, which surrounds its peptidoglycan layer. This is important clinically because certain antibiotics attack the peptidoglycan cell wall (e.g., penicillins) and are effective against gram-positive organisms, but are unable to penetrate the LPS-containing cell membrane of gram-negative organisms.

Several important organisms, including the *mycobacteria*, do not stain readily and therefore cannot be categorized by their uptake of stain using the Gram stain technique. However, these bacteria do take up the red stain *carbolfuchsin* and are therefore called **acid-fast** because they resist decolorization with acid alcohol and *retain their red stain*.

The *mycoplasma* (not to be confused with the mycobacteria just mentioned above) are another group of organisms that *have no cell wall* at all. These organisms are extremely small and cannot be classified as rods or cocci—they are **pleomorphic** due to their lack of a rigid cell wall. There are two pathogenic species of mycoplasma, discussed later.

B. Replication and Growth

Bacteria reproduce by **binary fission**, in which one parent cell divides to form two progeny cells, resulting in exponential growth. This cycle has four major phases (Fig. 1-2):

1. **Lag phase**—metabolic activity with no cell division.
2. **Log, or exponential, phase**—rapid cell division.
3. **Stationary phase**—nutrient depletion or toxic products cause growth to slow until a steady state between new cells and dying cells is achieved.
4. **Death phase**—decline in number of viable bacteria with associated prolonged phase of decline.

An organism's metabolism and growth are dependent on its *response to oxygen*. Clinically, bacterial specimens require incubation in an appropriate atmosphere for cell growth to occur. Most organisms require an adequate supply of oxygen for metabolism and growth, and are called **obligate aerobes**. However, some bacteria have the ability to utilize oxygen if it is present, but may also use the fermentation pathway in the absence of oxygen; these organisms are called **facultative anaerobes** (*Escherichia coli* is an example). Another subtype of bacteria is the **obligate anaerobes**, consisting of bacteria that cannot grow in the presence of oxygen because they lack enzymes that utilize and reduce oxygen (superoxide dismutase and catalase). If exposed to oxygen, some of these organisms may be killed rapidly, while others can survive but will not be able to grow. The final subtype is called **aerotolerant anaerobes**, which resemble facultative bacteria but have a fermentative metabolism both with and without an oxygen environment.

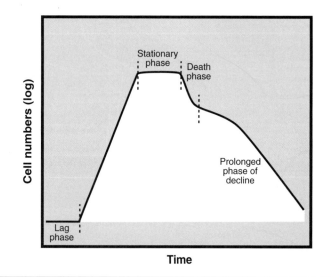

Figure 1–2 Bacterial growth phases.

C. Bacterium Overview

Gram-Positive Organisms (Fig. 1-3).

These organisms are easy to remember because there are only *seven main gram-positive bugs* that you need to know for Step 1. All the rest are gram-negative. The main gram-positive organisms are:

1. *S*taphylococcus
2. *S*treptococcus
3. *A*ctinomyces (often misclassified as a fungus!)
4. *B*acillus
5. *C*lostridium
6. *C*orynebacterium
7. *L*isteria

   ○ Remember the gram-positives by their first letters: *2 S's, A, B, 2 C's, and Listeria!* That's it!

- **Cocci:** The big two are *Staphylococci and Streptococci*. These organisms are differentiated clinically by the way they grow: *Staph grows in clusters* and *Strep grows in chains*.

   ○ Remember: **STREP** grows in a **STRIP**.

- *Staphylococci are catalase* +, meaning that they employ the enzyme catalase, which breaks down hydrogen peroxide (H_2O_2) into water and oxygen and results in bubbling. *Streptococci do not contain catalase*. Therefore, adding H_2O_2 to a bacterial colony can be used to differentiate between the two types of gram-positive bacteria.

   ○ Think of a cat walking with a cane (**staff**) to remember that *Staph* is **cat**alase-positive (Fig. 1-5).

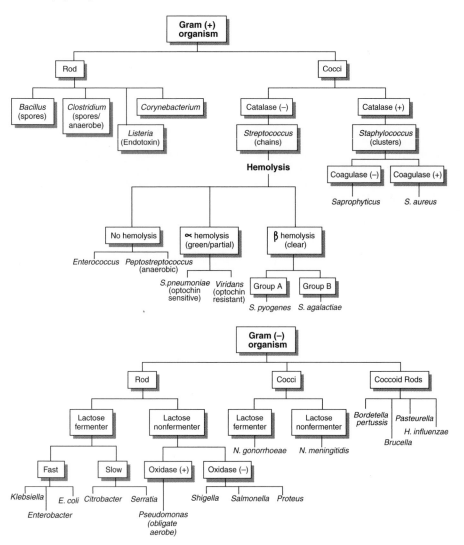

Figure 1–3 Laboratory algorithm for identifying gram-positive and gram-negative organisms. *Reprinted with permission from Neil O. Hardy, Westport, CT.*

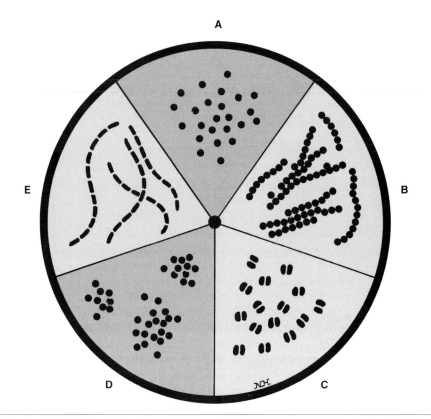

Figure 1–4 Appearance on staining of various bacteria under the microscope: **(A)** cocci, **(B)** streptococci, **(C)** diplococci, **(D)** staphylococci, **(E)** bacilli.

- To further differentiate the *Staph* species, a *coagulase test* can be used. *Staphylococcus aureus is the only staph species (that you need to know) that is coagulase-positive*! The enzyme coagulase activates prothrombin, causing blood to clot, and is tested by mixing plasma with a bacterial culture in a tube. *Staphylococcus aureus* will activate prothrombin in the plasma (via production of coagulase) and clots will form in the tube in 1 to 4 hours. In vivo, *Staph aureus* elaborates coagulase, which causes a protective fibrin shield to form around the organism protecting *Staph aureus* from the host immune system.

  ○ *Staphylococcus epidermidis* and *Staphylococcus saprophyticus* are *coagulase-negative*.

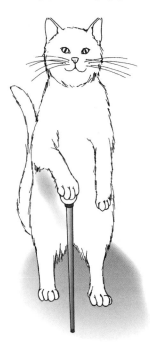

Figure 1–5 Remember that **Staph** is **cat**alase-positive.

TABLE 1-1	Lancefield Groups	
LANCEFIELD ANTIGEN	**ORGANISM**	**METABOLISM**
A	*Strep pyogenes*	Beta-hemolytic
B	*Strep agalactiae* (often called "group B strep" or "GBS")	Beta-hemolytic
D	*Enterococcus faecalis* *Strep bovis*	Alpha-, beta-, or gamma-hemolytic
(No letter)	*Strep viridans*	Alpha-hemolytic
(No letter)	*Strep pneumoniae*	Alpha-hemolytic

- One of the most important characteristics for ***streptococci identification*** is the type of hemolysis associated with the organism. *Alpha-hemolytic* streptococci produce the ***incomplete lysis of RBCs***, while *beta-hemolytic* streptococci are associated with the ***complete lysis of RBCs*** resulting from their production of the hemolysins, ***strepolysin O and S***. Beta-hemolytic streptococci are arranged into groups, known as **Lancefield groups**, on the basis of antigenic differences (Table 1-1).
- **Rods (Bacilli)**
    - **A** is for **Actinomyces**, which behaves like a fungus but actually is a gram-positive rod.
    - **B** is for **Bacillus** (*B. anthracis* and *B. cereus*)—both are **spore-formers**.
    - **C** is for **Corynebacterium** and **Clostridium**.
        - *Corynebacterium diphtheriae* is **pleomorphic** and resembles "Chinese letters" in a stained smear. *C. diphtheriae* forms a "pseudomembrane" in the pharynx and causes diphtheria.
        - *Clostridium* is a **spore-former** and has four important species: *C. botulinum, C. tetani, C. perfringens,* and *C. difficile.*
    - **D (no, actually L)** is for **Listeria**.
        - *L. monocytogenes* causes neonatal meningitis and gastroenteritis after ingestion of contaminated foods (especially soft cheeses).

Gram-Negative Organisms

There are many gram-negative organisms that cause disease in humans. It is easiest to remember them by the type of disease they cause, as outlined below and discussed in further detail throughout this book.

- **Cocci:** There is **only one gram-negative coccus to remember for Step 1**, and it is **Neisseria**. *Neisseria* has two important species, *N. meningitides* and *N. gonorrhoeae.*
    - *N. meningitidis* (aka "the meningococcus") causes meningitis and meningococcemia (with a classic petechial rash).
    - *N. gonorrhoeae* (aka "the gonococcus") causes gonorrhea and ophthalmia neonatorum when transmitted to a neonate during vaginal delivery.
- **Rods:**
    - *Cause gastrointestinal pathology:*
        - *Escherichia coli*—causes both watery and bloody diarrhea.
        - *Shigella dysenteriae*—results in bloody, mucoid diarrhea.
        - *Salmonella*—typhoidal and nontyphoidal disease.
        - *Vibrio cholerae*—transmitted fecal–orally after ingestion of contaminated water causes "rice water" diarrhea.
        - *Vibrio parahaemolyticus*—gastroenteritis after uncooked seafood (e.g., sushi and oysters).
        - *Helicobacter pylori*—causes duodenal ulcers and chronic gastritis.
    - *Cause genital-urinary disease:*
        - *Chlamydia trachomatis*—causes urethritis and PID and is the most common STD; also causes inclusion conjunctivitis in neonates.
        - *Gardnerella vaginalis*—causes bacterial vaginitis, or "BV"; produces "fishy odor"; slide reveals classic "clue cells."
        - *Haemophilus ducreyi*—causes STD chancroid, with painful genital ulcer and inguinal lymphadenopathy.
        - *Proteus mirabilis*—is urease splitting and causes UTI with staghorn calculus.

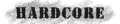

Beta-hemolytic organisms include *Strepococcus agalactiae, Staphylococcus aureus,* and *Listeria monocytogenes.*

HARDCORE

The only spore-forming organisms are the ***gram-positive rods***: *B. anthracis, C. perfringens,* and *C. tetani.*

- *Serratia*—causes UTIs in hospitalized patients; produces a red pigment.
- *Treponema pallidum*—a spirochete; causes syphilis. Subspecies of *T. pallidum* cause the nonvenereal diseases yaws, pinta, and bejel.

○ *Cause respiratory tract disease/pneumonia*:

- *Klebsiella pneumoniae*—associated with alcoholics.
- *Haemophilus influenzae*—causes acute epiglottitis and meningitis in kids; vaccinate with Hib vaccine; grow on chocolate agar.
- *Pseudomonas aeruginosa*—colonies are greenish-blue; causes infection in hospitalized or immunocompromised patients.
- *Bordatella pertussis*—causes whopping cough; grow on Bordet-Gengou agar.
- *Legionella pneumophila*—causes Legionnaires' pneumonia; grow on charcoal yeast agar.
- *Chlamydia pneumoniae*—causes atypical pneumonia in young adults.
- *Coxiella burnetti*—causes mild atypical pneumonia, aka "Q fever," after inhaling spores from wool or cowhides.

○ *Cause wound infection*:

- *Bacteroides fragilis*—an ANAEROBE that lives in the colon normally but can cause post-surgical abscesses and infection.

○ *Cause various diseases and are ZOONOTIC*:

- *Bartonella henselae*—causes cat-scratch disease in humans, characterized by fever and lymphadenopathy. Cats act as a reservoir.
- *Borrelia burgdorferi*—a spirochete; causes Lyme disease with classic "erythema chronicum migrans" rash after a bite from the *Ixodes* tick. Reservoir is the white-footed mouse and white-tailed deer.
- *Borrelia recurrentis*—a spirochete; causes relapsing fever after a bite from the human body louse *Pediculus humanus*. Reservoir is wild rodents.
- *Brucella abortus*—causes brucellosis, characterized by undulating fever and systemic disease. Causes abortions in cows; humans acquire the organism from infected animal meat or contacting infected animal placentas. Reservoir is cows.
- *Campylobacter jejuni*—causes diarrhea after ingestion of contaminated meat. Reservoir is pigs and chickens.
- *Chlamydia psittaci*—causes atypical pneumonia aka "psittacosis" after inhalation of dander from parrots. Reservoir is parrots and other birds.
- *Ehrlichia chaffeensis*—causes nonspecific feverish illness similar to RMSF without a rash after a bite from a tick. Reservoir is dogs.
- *Francisella tularensis*—causes tularemia, either in the form of a skin ulcer or pneumonia. Transmitted from handling infected rabbits. Reservoir is rabbits.
- *Leptospira interrogans*—a spirochete; causes leptospirosis with high fevers and muscle aches; can cause more severe Weil's disease. Transmitted by ingestion of urine from affected animals, such as by swimming in a urine-contaminated lake. Reservoir is dogs, cats, and livestock.
- *Pasteurella multocida*—causes wound infection following a cat scratch or bite. Reservoir is cats.
- *Rickettsia prowazekii*—causes EPIDEMIC typhus, with fever, headache, and rash, after bite from infected louse of flea. Reservoir is flying squirrels.
- *Rickettsia rickettsii*—causes Rocky Mountain spotted fever after a bite from the wood tick. Reservoir is wild rodents and rabbits.
- *Rickettsia typhi*—causes ENDEMIC typhus after bite from rat flea. Reservoir is rats.
- *Yersinia enterocolitica*—causes gastroenteritis following ingestion of water contaminated by feces of domestic animals, such as sheep or pigs. Reservoir is sheep and pigs.
- *Yersinia pestis*—causes bubonic plague via flea bite. Classic "bipolar stain" looks like a safety pin on Gram stain. Reservoir is rats.

Acid-Fast Organisms

There are *only three species* that you need to know for Step 1, and *all are rods*.

- **Rods:**
  ○ *Mycobacterium tuberculosis*—causes tuberculosis.
  ○ *Mycobacterium leprae*—causes leprosy. Cannot be grown on artificial media, but can grow in an armadillo (this organism's reservoir is the armadillo).
  ○ *Mycobacterium avium-intracellulare*—also called *Mycobacterium avium*-complex, or MAC. Causes severe multisystem organ dysfunction and bacteremia in AIDS patients.

Organisms with No Cell Wall: Mycoplasma

Remember, these are pleomorphic and *cannot be classified as rods or cocci*.

- *Mycoplasma pneumoniae*—causes atypical pneumonia, aka "walking pneumonia."
- *Ureaplasma urealyticum*—part of normal flora in most young, sexually active women. Commonly causes "nongonococcal urethritis" when it infects the lower urinary tract.

II. VIRUSES

For Step 1, you should remember which viruses are **DNA viruses** and which are **RNA viruses**, as well as which species of viruses come from the same *virus families*. It is easy to get caught up in viral names and the diseases they cause, but do not lose sight of the big picture! This overview should help you remember how to categorize the major viruses that you need know for Step 1 (Fig. 1-6).

A. DNA Viruses

There are only *six main DNA virus families* to remember, a **small heap** (*"HHeAPPP"*):

*HE*rpesviridae (enveloped)

*HE*padnaviridae (enveloped)

*A*denoviridae (naked)

*P*arvoviridae (naked)

*P*oxviridae (enveloped)

*P*apovaviridae (naked)

- Most DNA viruses are *double-stranded* and *replicate in the nucleus* of the host cell. There are *two DNA viruses that do not follow these generalizations*:

1. *Parvoviridae* is *single-stranded*.

   ○ Remember that "Parvus" means small! *Parvoviridae* is the smallest DNA virus, and thus only has room for one strand (not the usual two) of DNA.

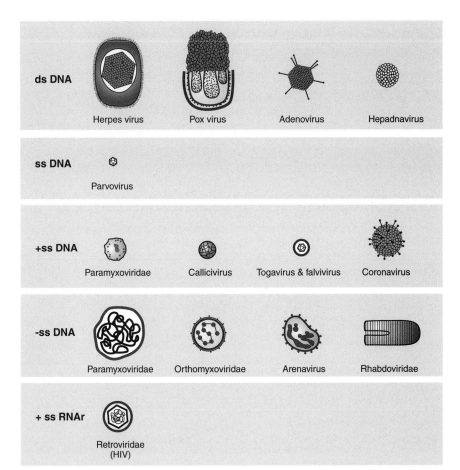

Figure 1–6 Overview of viral classification.

2. *Poxviridae replicates in the cytoplasm.*
   ○ *Poxviridae* is the most complex of all viruses. It has a large, *dumbbell-shaped genome* that codes for hundreds of proteins, including replication enzymes and structural proteins. Because it carries many of its own enzymes, *Poxviridae* does not need to pirate all host nuclear machinery for replication, and thus is able to replicate in the cytoplasm.

B. RNA Viruses

Most RNA viruses are *single-stranded and replicate in the cytoplasm.* Most are also *enveloped*, with three exceptions:

1. *Reoviridae* are *double-stranded.*
2. *Picornaviridae, Caliciviridae,* and *Reoviridae* do *not have envelopes* (they are naked).
3. *Retroviridae* and *Orthomyxoviridae replicate in the nucleus.*

- RNA viruses can be further classified by their *polarity.* The negative-polarity RNA viruses can be remembered by the mnemonic *BARF* and *PO(O)* (bodily functions that are generally regarded as *negative*):

  Bunyaviridae

  Arenaviridae

  Rhabdoviridae

  Filoviridae

  Paramyxoviridae

  Orthomyxoviridae

- The rest of the RNA viruses have positive polarity.

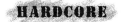

"Retro" means "reverse." Because the *Retroviridae* carry the enzyme *reverse transcriptase*, they can convert viral RNA into DNA, which integrates into the host genome's DNA.

III. FUNGI

There are two major forms of fungi, **molds** (also called *Mycelia*) and **yeasts**.

- Molds are *multicellular*, and colonies are made up of threadlike hyphae that look like the branches of a tree.
  ○ Molds *reproduce by forming spores.*
- Yeasts are *unicellular* and can form long chains of yeast cells called *pseudohyphae.*
  ○ Yeasts *reproduce by budding.*
- Some fungi can grow as either a yeast or a mold, depending on temperature. These fungi are called **dimorphic fungi**.
  ○ *Sporothrix schenckii*—"rose gardener's disease."
  ○ *Candida albicans*—oval-budding yeast diagnosed with KOH stain.
  ○ *Cryptococcus*—found in pigeon droppings, affects primarily the immunocompromised.
  ○ *Histoplasma*—found in Mississippi and Ohio River basins.
  ○ *Paracoccidioides*—results in painful ulcerated mouth lesions.

IV. PATHOGENICITY OF MICROORGANISMS

Medical microbiology is essentially the study of microbial pathogenicity, or the capacity of an infectious organism to cause disease. The term *virulence* refers to the degree of an organism's pathogenicity measured by the number of organisms required to cause disease and is dependent on that organism's *virulence factors.* Virulence factors are specific structures or capabilities of microbial organisms that enable that organism to cause pathology. Virulence factors are heavily tested on Step 1 and are important for understanding each organism's potential for causing disease (Fig. 1-7).

A. Life-Cycles

Many microbial organisms have developed complex life-cycles that *facilitate transmission and cell survival.* These life-cycles typically involve a **vector**, which is another organism that transmits the infectious organism to humans. Humans can also become infected as an accidental host in certain organism life-cycles.

B. Sources of Infection

Obligate pathogens are always associated with a disease, while organisms that make up the normal flora only invade under specific or abnormal circumstances. Often, alteration of the environment will increase the risk of disease.

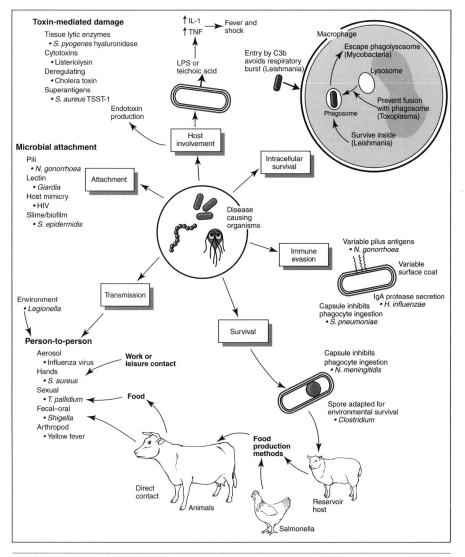

Figure 1–7 Pathogenicity of microorganisms.

- **Normal flora**—the body contains many resident microorganisms that protect the host by competing with pathogens for colonization sites. Remember that antibiotics suppress the normal flora and may allow colonization and infection by naturally resistant organisms (Table 1-2).

C. Virulence Factors

Toxins

Toxins are some of the most lethal and heavily tested categories of virulence factors. Toxins are unique to bacteria and consist of two general types: *endotoxins* and *exotoxins*.

- **Endotoxins** are derived from integral components of the cell wall (lipopolysaccharide) of *gram-negative bacteria* (such as meningococci). The exception is *Listeria*, which is a gram-positive organism that *has an endotoxin*, but no exotoxin.
    - Endotoxins possess *low toxicity*, but may cause septic shock (TNF and IL-1 activation).
    - Endotoxins result in the generalized effects of fever and shock.
    - The toxic portion of the endotoxin LPS molecule is *lipid A*.
    - Endotoxins have poor antigenicity.
    - Endotoxins are *heat stable*—will remain stable at 100°C for up to 1 hour.
    - No vaccines are currently available for endotoxins.
- **Exotoxins** are secreted from certain gram-positive and gram-negative organisms (such as *Clostridium, Corynebacterium diphtheriae,* and *Staphylococcus aureus*—Table 1-3).
    - Exotoxins possess high toxicity: *more rapidly destructive than endotoxin.*

TABLE 1-2	Normal Flora
TISSUE	**ORGANISMS**
Nasopharynx	*Streptococci viridans* (mouth)
	Staphylococcus aureus (nose)
	Corynebacterium (nose)
	Haemophilus
	Neisseria
	Fusobacterium
	Eikenella corrodens
	Actinomyces
Skin	*Staphylococcus*
	Streptococcus
	Corynebacterium
	Candida albicans
Upper bowel	*Enterococcus*
	Candida albicans
Lower bowel	*Bacteroides*
	Clostridium
	Peptostreptococcus
Vagina	*Lactobaccilus*
	Streptococcus
	Corynebacterium
	Candida albicans
	Actinomyces

○ *Neurotoxins* (e.g., tetanus, botulinum) and *enterotoxins* are each types of exotoxins.

○ Enterotoxins act on the GI tract to cause diarrhea by increasing the osmotic pull of fluid into the intestine by three mechanisms: the inhibition of NaCl resorption, the destruction of intestinal epithelial cells, and the activation of host intestinal secretion.

○ Exposure to exotoxins results in the formation of host antitoxins.

○ Structurally, many exotoxins possess an *A-B subunit* structure, in which the *A (active)* subunit possesses the toxic activity and the *B (binding)* subunit acts to bind the exotoxin to specific receptors on host cell membranes. The A subunit commonly acts by ADP-ribosylation, which can either inactivate or hyperactivate the target protein, causing a varying spectrum of pathology between organisms. Important A-B exotoxins include diphtheria toxin, tetanus toxin, botulinum toxin, cholera toxin, and *E. coli* enterotoxin.

○ Exotoxins are *heat labile*—rapidly destroyed at 60°C.

○ Toxoids may be used as vaccines.

Adherence to Host Cell Surfaces

Invading organisms must *attach themselves to host tissues to colonize the body*. Each bug has a unique capacity to bind various tissues using specialized structures such as pili, capsules, and glycocalyces.

- *Pili*—Rigid surface appendages that mediate attachment of the organism to epithelium, typically urinary tract epithelium (*N. gonorrhoeae*, *S. pyogenes*, and *E. coli*).
  - ○ Another class of pili (sex pili) is involved in the attachment of donor and recipient bacteria in conjugation.
  - ○ Pili can also confer antiphagocytic properties, such as the M protein of *S. pyogenes*.
- *Glycocalyx*—A loose network of polysaccharide fibrils that surrounds certain bacterial cell walls and is associated with the adhesive properties of bacterial cell walls.
  - ○ Glycocalyx allows *S. epidermidis* to adhere to the endothelium of heart valves.

Environmental Survival

Spores are structures that enable certain gram-positive bacteria (*B. anthracis*, *C. perfringens*, and *C. tetani*) to survive in unfavorable environmental conditions such as desiccation, heat, and various chemicals (helminth eggs act in a similar capacity).

- Endospores are formed as a survival response to specific adverse nutritional conditions.
- Spores are metabolically inactive.

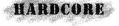

The A subunit of many A-B subunit exotoxins targets elongation factor-2 (EF-2), resulting in the inhibition of protein synthesis.

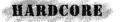

Although exotoxins consist of proteins released from bacterial cells, endotoxins exist as normal components of the gram-negative cell wall that "slough off" during cell lysis (destruction). Endotoxin release may lead to bacteremia, sepsis, and septic shock (endotoxic shock). There are no specific endotoxin names to memorize, but be familiar with the exotoxins in Table 1-3.

- These structures germinate under favorable nutritional conditions.
- Spores are not reproductive structures.

Invasion and Immune Evasion

Microorganisms are constantly being attacked by the immune system after gaining access to the human body (except in the immunocompromised host) and must overcome the human immune defense to survive. Microorganisms possess several defense mechanisms that protect themselves:

- *Coagulase*—enzyme that accelerates the formation of a fibrin clot, which walls off the infected area and protects the bug from phagocytosis (S. *aureus*).
- *Leukocidins*—enzyme that can destroy neutrophilic leukocytes and macrophages.
- *IgA proteases*—enzyme that degrade host immunoglobulin IgA and allows the organism to adhere to mucous membranes (N. *gonorrhoeae*, H. *influenzae*, S. *pneumoniae*).
- *Polysaccharide capsule*—prevents host phagocytes from adhering to the bacteria (S. *pneumoniae*, N. *meningitidis*, H. *influenzae*).
- *Cell wall proteins*—M protein and protein A. The M protein of S. *pyogenes* is antiphagocytic, while the protein A of S. *aureus* functions by binding to IgG and preventing the activation of complement.
- *Intracellular survival*—allows organisms to sneak past the circulating immunocells.
- *Lipopolysaccharide* of gram-negative cell walls, which makes them resistant to host complement. LPS is negatively charged and consists of lipid A, polysaccharide unit, and long-chain fatty acids. LPS is a target of innate immunity and contains major surface antigenic determinants including O antigen in the polysaccharide units.

TABLE 1-3	Commonly Tested Exotoxins		
TOXINS	**ORGANISM**	**MECHANISM**	**DISEASE**
Enterotoxins			
Choleragen	*Vibrio cholerae*	A-B subunit structure. Binds GM1 gangliosides on intestinal cell membranes, increasing cAMP levels that result in increased intraluminal NaCl. This fluids and electrolytes into the gut pulls	Cholera—severe watery diarrhea and dehydration
Shigella toxin	*Shigella dysenteriae* EHEC EIEC (*E. coli* releases *Shigella*-like toxin)	Binds intestinal epithelial cells, inhibits protein synthesis by inactivating the 60S ribosomal subunit	Bloody, mucoid diarrhea
E. coli heat-labile toxin	*E. coli* *Camplyobacter jejuni* *Bacillus cereus*	Similar to choleragen: binds GM1 gangliosides on intestinal cell membranes, increasing cAMP levels and resulting in increased intraluminal NaCl. This pulls fluids and electrolytes into the gut	Diarrhea
E. coli heat-stable toxin	*E. coli*	Binds intestinal brush boarder, activating guanylate cyclase to increase cGMP (inhibits resorption of NaCl and increases osmotic pull of fluid/electrolytes into the gut)	Diarrhea
Staphylococcal heat-stable toxin	*Staphylococcus aureus* *Bacillus cereus* (heat-stable toxin)	Binds intestinal brush boarder, increases cGMP inhibiting resorption of NaCl and increasing osmotic pull of fluid/electrolytes into the gut	These infections are caused by ingestion of the enterotoxin in contaminated food, rather than the local release into the GI tract as with other causes of infectious diarrhea. Results in diarrhea and vomiting lasting less than 24 hours (*B. cereus* poisoning is characterized by vomiting with limited diarrhea)
Neurotoxins			
Botulinum toxin	*Clostridium botulinum*	A-B subunit structure. Inhibits acetylcholine release from motor end-plates at NMJ	Flaccid paralysis
Tetanus toxin	*Clostridium tetani*	A-B subunit structure. Binds neuronal gangliosides and blocks the release of inhibitory neurotransmitters	Uncontrolled muscle contractions (lockjaw)
Tissue-Invasive Toxins			
Hyaluronidase	*Streptococcus pyogenes*	Breaks down proteoglycans	Abscess formation with systemic infection
Hemolysins Streptolysin O and S	*Streptococcus pyogenes*	Hemolyzes RBCs	Abscess formation with systemic infection

(Continued)

TABLE 1-3	Commonly Tested Exotoxins (cont.)		
TOXINS	**ORGANISM**	**MECHANISM**	**DISEASE**
Streptokinase	*Streptococcus pyogenes*	Activates plasminogen (lyses fibrin clots)	Abscess formation with systemic infection
DNase	*Streptococcus pyogenes*	Hydrolyzes DNA	Abscess formation with systemic infection
RNase	*Streptococcus pyogenes*	Hydrolyzes RNA	Abscess formation with systemic infection
Lipases	*Staphylococcus aureus*	Hydrolyzes lipids	Abscess formation with systemic infection
Staphylokinase	*Staphylococcus aureus*	Activates plasminogen (lyses fibrin clots)	Abscess formation with systemic infection
Leukocidin	*Staphylococcus aureus*	Lyses WBCs	Abscess formation with systemic infection
Exfoliatin	*Staphylococcus aureus*	Lyses epithelial cells	Scalded skin syndrome in infants
Penicillinase	*Staphylococcus aureus*	Destroys penicillins	Abscess formation with systemic infection
Alpha toxin	*Clostridium perfringens*	Hydrolyzes lecithin in cell membranes (causes cell death)	Gas gangrene
Pyogenic Toxins			
Toxic-shock syndrome toxin	*Staphylococcus aureus*	Activates cytokines, specifically IL-1	Sepsis
Streptococcus pyrogenic toxin	*Streptococcus pyogenes* (Group A *Streptococcus*)	Activates cytokines, specifically IL-1	Scarlet fever
Miscellaneous Toxins			
Lethal factor	*Bacillus anthracis*	Kills macrophages	Anthrax
Edema factor	*Bacillus anthracis*	Increases cAMP and inhibits phagocytosis	Anthrax
Protective antigen	*Bacillus anthracis*	Allows EF entry into cells	Anthrax
C. difficile toxin A and B	*Clostridium difficile*	Toxin A increases fluid secretion and inflammation. Toxin B is cytotoxic to colonic epithelial cells	Pseudomembranous enterocolitis
Diptheriae toxin	*Corynebacterium diptheriae*	A-B subunit structure. ADP ribosylates elongation-factor (EF-2). Inhibits translation of human mRNA	Diphtheria
Pertussis toxin	*Bordetella pertussis*	Activates membrane G-proteins, activating adenylate cyclase leading to the inhibition of neutrophils and MACs	Whooping cough
Pseudomonas exotoxin A	*Pseudomonas aeruginosa*	Inhibits protein synthesis by inhibiting EF-2 (same mechanism as diphtheria)	Clinical *Pseudomonas* infection

CHAPTER 2

Infections of Neonates, Infants, and Children

Bugs discussed in this chapter:

- *Staphylococcus aureus*
- *Streptococcus pneumoniae*
- *Streptococcus agalactiae:* Group B *Streptococcus* (GBS)
- *Listeria monocytogenes*
- *Haemophilus influenzae*
- *Neisseria meningitides*
- *Streptococcus pyogenes*
- *Streptococcus pneumonae*
- *Corynebacterium diphtheriae*
- *Bordetella pertussis*
- *Chlamydia trachomatis*
- *Mycoplasma pneumoniae*
- Parainfluenza virus
- Influenza A and B virus

- *Adenovirus*
- Respiratory syncytial virus
- Parvovirus B 19
- Human herpesvirus 6
- Measles virus
- Mumps virus
- Varicella-zoster virus
- *Clostridium botulinum*
- *Shigella dysenteriae*
- *Rotovirus*
- *Adenovirus*
- *Enterobius vermicularis*
- *Molluscum contagiosum*
- Tinea
- *Pseudomonas aeruginosa*

I. CENTRAL NERVOUS SYSTEM

Meningitis refers to the inflammation of the meninges (the tissues that surround the brain or spinal cord). This diagnosis cannot be missed in infants because of its potentially fatal complications. These little patients may present as irritable and febrile with paradoxical crying (increased crying or fussiness when held). Older children present with headache, neck pain, and nuchal rigidity. Diagnosis is made by obtaining cerebral spinal fluid (CSF) via lumbar puncture for culture and cytology study (Table 2-1).

A. Gram-Positive Bacteria

Listeria monocytogenes

- Facultative-intracellular gram-positive bacillus
- Catalase +
- Facultative anaerobe

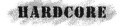

HARDCORE

The CSF from children with bacterial meningitis will have >100 polymorphonuclear leukocytes, glucose concentration <50, and elevated protein concentration.

TABLE 2-1	Cerebral Spinal Fluid Analysis for Infectious Etiologies		
	BACTERIAL	**VIRAL**	**MYCOBACTERIAL/FUNGAL**
Protein	↑	↔	↑
Glucose	↓	↔	↓
Lymphs	↑ (PMNs)	↑ (Lymphocytes)	↑ (Lymphocytes)
Pressure	↑	↔	↔/↑

CLINICAL CORRELATES—NEWBORN MENINGITIS

➤ *Listeria* meningitis most often occurs in neonates *over 3 days of age*. After invading the bloodstream, *Listeria* has a tropism for the CSF and deep brain structures and can result in meningitis.

➤ The typical reservoir for *Listeria* is dairy products, and it can colonize the gastrointestinal tract without causing symptoms.

Streptococcus agalactiae: Group B *Streptococcus*

- Gram-positive coccus in chains
- Group B, beta-hemolytic
- Facultative anaerobe

CLINICAL CORRELATES—NEWBORN AND INFANT MENINGITIS

➤ GBS infection is the *most common cause of meningitis in newborns and infants*. Infection most commonly occurs during birth when a neonate passes through the vagina of a woman colonized by GBS (30% to 40% of all pregnant women are normally colonized).

  - Group **B** is for **B**abies

Streptococcus pneumoniae

- Gram-positive, lancet-shaped diplococcus in chains
- Catalase –
- Ferments inulin
- Optochin-sensitive (+ Quellung reaction)
- Alpha-hemolytic

CLINICAL CORRELATES—MENINGITIS IN CHILDREN (1 MONTH TO 2 YEARS OLD) AND ADULTS

➤ Central *S. pneumoniae* invasion resulting in meningitis may progress from a peripheral infection such as otitis media or sinusitis. Once in the CSF, these bacteria promote inflammation, alter vascular permeability, and induce the influx of leukocytes resulting in brain edema and inflammation.

➤ *S. pneumoniae* is optochin sensitive and encapsulated, resulting in a positive Quellung reaction.

B. Gram-Negative Bacteria

Haemophilus influenzae

- Gram-negative rod
- Oxidase +
- Non-lactose fermenter
- Aerobe

CLINICAL CORRELATES—MENINGITIS IN KIDS BETWEEN 2 AND 18 YEARS OLD

➤ Before standardized vaccinations for this bug, *H. influenzae* type B was the major cause of bacterial meningitis in children. Although the incidence of infection has markedly decreased, keep this bug in the differential for the board exam.

➤ The *H. influenzae* vaccine contains type b capsular polysaccharide conjugated to diphtheria toxoid and is typically administered between 2 and 18 months of age.

Neisseria meningitidis ("Meningococcus")

- Gram-negative diplococci
- Ferments maltose and glucose
- Oxidase +
- Anaerobe

CLINICAL CORRELATES—MENINGITIS IN CHILDREN AND YOUNG ADULTS

➤ *N. meningitidis* is the *leading cause of bacterial meningitis in children and young adults*. *N. meningitidis* meningitis typically occurs in late winter and presents with the standard onset of fever, nausea, vomiting, headache, and nuchal rigidity. This infection *progresses rapidly* and can transition from mild to severe and fatal disease in a matter of hours.

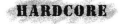

GBS (+) pregnant women should be prophylactically treated with penicillin before delivery.

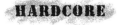

In addition to being the most frequent cause of meningitis in children, *S. pneumoniae* is also the leading cause of meningitis in adults.

HARDCORE

H. influenzae does not cause influenza (influenza virus does).

➤ Possesses a capsular polysaccharide that inhibits phagocytosis, an IgA protease that degrades IgA, and a LPS that can cause extensive tissue necrosis, intravascular coagulation, hemorrhage, and shock.

➤ Identify *N. meningitides* with **positive CSF oxidase test and cultures**.

II. PULMONARY

A. Gram-Positive Bacteria

Corynebacterium diphtheriae

- Gram-positive rod
- Catalase +
- Anaerobe
- Non-spore forming

CLINICAL CORRELATES—PSEUDOMEMBRANOUS PHARYNGITIS

➤ *Corynebacterium diphtheriae* has become an uncommon cause of child pharyngitis in developed countries since the **DTaP (or DPT) vaccine** became commonplace. However, if this bug does surface, it can have fatal consequences. The most important clinical feature of infection with *C. diphtheriae* is the development of areas of white exudates that coalesce to form an **adherent gray pseudomembrane that bleeds with scraping**.

➤ Diptheria toxin (beta-prophage) inhibits the translation of human mRNA by **inhibiting EF-2 via ADP ribosylation**.

Streptococcus agalactiae (Group B Streptococcus)

- Gram-positive coccus in chains
- Group B, beta-hemolytic
- Facultative anaerobe

CLINICAL CORRELATES—NEWBORN PNEUMONIA

➤ GBS is the **most common cause of early-onset newborn pneumonia**. GBS bugs injure lung epithelial cells with beta-hemolysin, leading to alveolar edema and hemorrhage.

Streptococcus pneumoniae

- Gram-positive coccus in chains
- Catalase –
- Ferments inulin
- Optochin-sensitive (+ Quellung reaction)
- Alpha-hemolytic

CLINICAL CORRELATES—COMMUNITY-ACQUIRED PNEUMONIA (LOBAR)

➤ Pneumococci are aerosolized from the nasopharynx to the alveolus, where they can cause the classic **lobar bacterial pneumonia**. *Pneumococcus* is a typical cause of community-acquired pneumonia and the most common cause of invasive bacterial infection in children.

Streptococcus pyogenes

- Gram-positive cocci in chains
- Catalase –
- Group A Lancefield
- Facultative anaerobe

CLINICAL CORRELATES—BACTERIAL PHARYNGITIS (STREP THROAT), SCARLET FEVER, RHEUMATIC FEVER, POSTSTREPTOCOCCAL GLOMERULONEPHRITIS

➤ *S. pyogenes* is the **most frequent cause of acute bacterial pharyngitis in children**. "Strep throat" is associated with severe, purulent inflammation of the oropharynx and tonsils.

➤ Acutely, *S. pyogenes* infection can develop into **scarlet fever**, which is an **erythrogenic toxin-induced vasodilation** that presents as an extensive morbilliform erythematous rash, desquamation and peeling of fingertips, and a "strawberry tongue." These patients will have an **elevated antistreptolysin O (ASO) titer**.

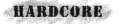

HARDCORE

Patients with menigococcus may have a **petechial rash** on the trunk and lower portions of the body.

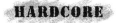

HARDCORE

H. meningitidis is the **second most common cause of adult bacterial meningitis** (behind *S. pneumoniae*).

HARDCORE

Widespread *N. menigitidis* infections have been associated with **military recruits**.

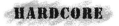

HARDCORE

Avoid scraping the pseudomembrane of diphtheria because this may precipitate bleeding and compromise the airway.

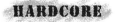

HARDCORE

C. diphtheriae occur in V- and L-shaped arrangements on **tellurite agar** that appear club shaped and similar to "**Chinese characters**."

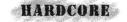

HARDCORE

The DTaP vaccine protects against **D**iphtheria, **T**etanus, and **P**ertussis.

HARDCORE

Rheumatic heart disease is the major cause of acquired valvular disease in the world.

HARDCORE

The **JONES criteria** describe symptoms of acute rheumatic fever:

J – joints (arthritis)

O – obvious (carditis)

N – nodules (subcutaneous)

E – erythema marginatum

S – syndenham's chorea

➤ **Acute rheumatic fever (ARF)** is an autoimmune disorder that can follow an episode of acute *S. pyogenes* pharyngitis. Several weeks after the initial pharyngitis, the patient presents with arthritis, carditis, chorea, subcutaneous nodules, or **erythema marginatum** (a pink nonpruritic rash that affects only the trunk or limbs, but not the face). Patients with acute rheumatic fever are at risk for developing **rheumatic heart disease (RHD)**, which occurs 10 to 20 years after the original presentation of ARF and manifests as *heart valve damage and carditis*. Most commonly, the mitral valve is affected resulting in mitral stenosis.

➤ **Poststreptococcal glomerulonephritis** is another potential sequela of *S. pyogenes* pharyngitis. This disease is initiated by antigen-antibody complexes that deposit on the glomerular basement membrane. The clinical presentation can vary from asymptomatic, microscopic hematuria to a full-blown acute nephritic syndrome, characterized by red to brown urine, proteinuria (which can reach the nephrotic range), edema, hypertension, and acute renal failure.

B. Gram-Negative Bacteria

Bordetella pertussis

- Gram-negative coccobacillus
- Aerobic

CLINICAL CORRELATES—WHOOPING COUGH

➤ *B. pertussis* causes the infamous **"whooping cough,"** a respiratory illness characterized by paroxysmal coughing that follows a forced inspiratory effort and results in a "whooping" sound. This disease occurs in three stages:

1. **Catarrhal stage**—appears similar to the "common cold," with mild cough and coryza, and generally lasts 1 to 2 weeks. Instead of improving like a typical upper respiratory infection (URI), the cough gradually increases.

2. **Paroxysmal stage**—coughing persists and the severity increases, occurring in paroxysmal attacks of a long series of coughs during which the child may develop gagging and cyanosis and appears to be struggling for breath. This stage may last 6 to 12 weeks.

3. **Convalescent stage**—the cough continues to decrease gradually over several weeks to months.

Chlamydia trachomatis

- Gram-negative
- Obligate intracellular parasite

CLINICAL CORRELATES—ATYPICAL PNEUMONIA

➤ *C. trachomatis* initially infects newborns during their passage through an infected birth canal, but presents between 4 and 11 weeks of age. Infants with *Chlamydia* pneumonia develop tachypnea and a *staccato cough*, but have minimal fever, resulting in the common name of **afebrile pneumonia**.

HARDCORE

M. pneumoniae's lack of a cell wall causes the mycoplasma to have a "*fried egg*" appearance.

HARDCORE

Diagnosis of *M. pneumoniae* pneumonia is based on *cold agglutinin titers* that measure IgM antibodies.

- IgM = *I'M cold*

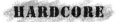

HARDCORE

The most common respiratory illnesses in children are:

1. RSV
2. Parainfluenza (croup)
3. Rhinovirus
4. Adenovirus

C. Mycoplasma

Mycoplasma pneumoniae

- Pleomorphic
- No cell wall

CLINICAL CORRELATES—COMMUNITY-ACQUIRED PNEUMONIA

➤ Atypical, or "*walking*" pneumonia caused by *Mycoplasma pneumoniae* presents abruptly with fever, malaise and myalgia, and a gradually worsening, nonproductive cough despite the improvement of other symptoms.

➤ Chest X-ray will demonstrate an *infiltrative pattern that looks much worse than the clinical scenario*.

D. Viruses

Adenovirus

- Double-stranded DNA
- Naked virus
- Icosahedral nucleocapsid

CLINICAL CORRELATES—UPPER RESPIRATORY TRACT INFECTION

➤ Adenoviruses are an important cause of febrile illnesses in young children. They are most frequently associated with upper respiratory tract syndromes such as pharyngitis or coryza, but can also cause pneumonia, as well as gastrointestinal, ophthalmologic, genitourinary, and neurologic diseases.

➤ Adenovirus infections are prevalent in *daycare centers and in households with young children* in which transmission occurs via aerosol droplets, fecal–oral, and contact with contaminated fomites.

Human Herpesvirus 6

- Double-stranded, DNA virus
- Gamma herpesvirus
- Icosahedral nucleocapsid

CLINICAL CORRELATES—ROSEOLA INFANTUM

➤ Roseola is an illness of children younger than 2 years that classically begins with a *high fever* (may be in excess of 40°C) lasting 3 to 5 days. Even during the fever, most children appear well, active, and alert. *As the child's fever subsides, a blanching macular or maculopapular rash develops*, starting on the neck and trunk and spreading to the face and extremities. The rash usually persists for 1 to 2 days and is self-limiting.

  ▪ *Remember*—the rash of roseola is like a "**rose**" that blooms **after** a high fever.

Influenza A and B Virus

- Negative, single-stranded, RNA virus
- Orthomyxovirus

CLINICAL CORRELATES—TYPICAL PNEUMONIA

➤ Influenza is spread by respiratory droplets and infects respiratory epithelial cells, presenting as an acute but typically self-limited and uncomplicated disease. The most common complications of influenza in children are *lower respiratory tract involvement and otitis media*.

Parainfluenza Virus

- Negative, single-stranded RNA virus
- *Paramyxoviridae*

CLINICAL CORRELATES—CROUP, LOWER RESPIRATORY TRACT INFECTIONS

➤ Croup is a respiratory illness characterized by inspiratory stridor, cough, and hoarseness resulting from inflammation in the larynx and subglottic airway. A *barking cough* is the hallmark of a croup infection.

➤ In infants and young children, parainfluenza virus is second to respiratory syncytial virus (RSV) as the leading cause of *acute lower respiratory tract infections*. Parainfluenza virus initially infects epithelial cells of the nose and oropharynx before spreading distally to the large and small airways.

Parvovirus B 19

- Single-stranded, DNA virus
- *Parvoviridae*
- Icosahedral nucleocapsid

CLINICAL CORRELATES—ERYTHEMA INFECTIOSUM (FIFTH DISEASE)

➤ Erythema infectiosum, or *fifth disease*, often occurs in outbreaks among school-aged children and is characterized by a malar, erythematous rash that appears on the face (the so-called **slapped cheek rash**), as well as a reticulated or lacelike rash on the trunk and extremities. By the time the rash develops, a child with fifth disease typically feels well and acts normally.

Respiratory Syncytial Virus

- Negative, single-stranded RNA virus
- Paramyxovirus

CLINICAL CORRELATES—UPPER AND LOWER RESPIRATORY TRACT INFECTION

➤ RSV is the *most common cause of lower respiratory tract infection in children younger than 1 year*. RSV causes seasonal outbreaks (wintertime) in which individuals infected with RSV develop cough,

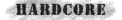

HARDCORE

Roseola may be complicated with thrombocytopenia from bone marrow suppression.

HARDCORE

Influenza infection is associated with Guillain Barré syndrome (ascending paralysis) in adults, and Reye's syndrome in children (from the concurrent use of aspirin) that results in acute encephalopathy.

HARDCORE

Parainfluenza consists of four major serotypes of human PIV (PIV-1, 2, 3, 4). PIV-1 is the leading cause of croup in children.

HARDCORE

Fifth disease, arthropathy, and nonimmune hydrops fetalis are clinical presentations linked to B-19 infection.

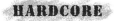

HARDCORE

Parvovirus B 19 is associated with *splenic crisis in patients with sickle cell disease*.

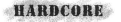

HARDCORE

Parvovirus is the smallest DNA virus.

coryza, rhinorrhea, conjunctivitis, and otitis media. In healthy individuals this disease is self-limiting.

➤ Transmission of RSV occurs via *direct contact of virus-containing secretions* onto nasopharyngeal or ocular mucous membranes.

III. OTHER IMPORTANT PEDIATRIC VIRAL INFECTIONS

Measles Virus
- Negative, single-stranded RNA virus
- Paramyxovirus

CLINICAL CORRELATES—MEASLES (RUBEOLA)

➤ Measles infection occurs in four stages: *incubation, prodrome, exanthem, and recovery*. During prodrome, patients typically suffer from fever, conjunctivitis, coryza, and cough, as well as the development of an exanthem known as **Koplik's spots**. Koplik's spots are small whitish, grayish, or bluish spots seen on the buccal mucosa that have been described as *"grains of salt on a red background."* Following the prodrome is an exanthem stage characterized by a blanching, maculopapular rash with *cranial-to-caudal progression*. This lasts for about 48 hours and is followed by the recovery period (Fig 2-1).

Mumps Virus
- Negative, single-stranded RNA virus
- Paramyxovirus

CLINICAL CORRELATES—MUMPS

➤ Mumps infection begins as a nonspecific prodrome consisting of low-grade fever, headache, myalgias, and anorexia. These symptoms are generally followed by the development of **parotitis**, a classic feature of mumps infection. **Mumps orchitis** is another complication characterized by an abrupt onset of fever, severe testicular pain, and swelling and erythema of the scrotum.

Varicella-Zoster Virus (Human Herpesvirus 3)
- Double-stranded, DNA virus
- Herpesvirus alpha
- Icosahedral nucleocapsid

CLINICAL CORRELATES—VARICELLA (CHICKENPOX)

➤ The chickenpox rash appears in successive *crops of vesicles* over a 3- to 4-day period. These lesions are pruritic and consist of a pustular component that eventually crusts over. These lesions *appear in different stages of development* on the face, trunk, and extremities. New lesion formation generally stops within 4 days, and most lesions have fully crusted by day 6.

HARDCORE

Think of RSV infection in a child <1 year old with tachypnea, wheeze, and URI symptoms.

HARDCORE

Measles triad: cough, coryza, conjunctivitis.

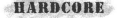

HARDCORE

Mumps diagnosis involves isolating the mumps virus, identifying a significant rise in IgG titers, or isolating positive IgM mumps antibodies.

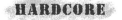

HARDCORE

Mumps infection is now rarely seen due to routine vaccination with the MMR vaccine.

HARDCORE

There is *no association* between mumps orchitis and the development of testicular cancer, but if orchitis occurs bilaterally it can result in *sterility*.

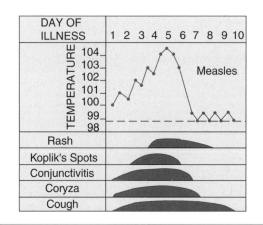

Figure 2–1 Measles, an acute exanthem characterized by rash. *LifeART image copyright © 2006 Lippincott Williams & Wilkins. All rights reserved.*

➤ Transmission of the varicella-zoster virus occurs via *direct cutaneous contact* with vesicle fluid from skin lesions or from *aerosolized droplets* from nasopharyngeal secretions of an infected individual.

➤ Diagnosis occurs by Tzanck smear or fluorescent antibody staining.

IV. GASTROINTESTINAL

A. Bacteria

Clostridium botulinum
- Gram-positive rod
- Anaerobe
- Endospores

CLINICAL CORRELATES—BOTULISM
➤ Botulism may occur in infants following ingestion of spores. On the board exam, this generally occurs after an infant is given *honey*. *C. botulinum*'s *preformed exotoxin* causes generalized weakness and a loss of head and limb control that results in a **floppy-baby appearance**.
- **Remember:** Clostridium *lives in a closet* and *gets no air* (an anaerobe).

B. Parasites

Enterobius vermicularis
- Helminth

CLINICAL CORRELATES—PINWORM INFECTION
➤ Pinworm infections occur most frequently in school children aged 5 to 10 years old and are characterized by intense *night time perianal itching* (pruritus ani).

➤ Transmission of *Enterobius vermicularis* occurs via direct anus-to-mouth spread. Following ingestion, the eggs hatch and release larvae within the intestine. Larvae develop into adult worms over several week, and then migrate out through the rectum *onto the perianal skin to deposit eggs*. This usually occurs at night, causing an inflammatory reaction to the presence of adult worms and eggs on the perianal skin. As the child scratches, eggs get lodged under the fingernails and transmission can occur.

➤ Diagnosis is made by the *"Scotch tape" test*, which is performed by sticking clear Scotch tape against the perianal skin. The eggs will stick to the tape and can then be visualized.

C. Viruses

Adenovirus
- Double-stranded DNA
- Naked virus
- Icosahedral nucleocapsid

CLINICAL CORRELATES—INFANT DIARRHEA
➤ Although rotavirus-associated diarrhea is more common, enteric adenoviruses can also cause prolonged diarrheal syndromes in infants, especially in group settings such as *day-care centers*. Viral culture is the most sensitive and specific method for detection.

Rotavirus
- Double-stranded, DNA virus
- Reovirus

CLINICAL CORRELATES—DIARRHEA
➤ Rotaviruses are the most important cause of *viral gastroenteritis* and are the most common cause of fatal diarrhea in children.

➤ Rotavirus is diagnosed with ELISA.
- Rotavirus is like a *"rota-rooter"* to the GI tract, resulting in diarrhea.

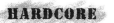

HARDCORE

After gaining entry to the host cell, the varicella-zoster virus undergoes localized replication that is followed by an incubation phase lasting about 15 days.

HARDCORE

A person is considered infectious with chickenpox from 48 hours prior to the onset of rash until all skin lesions have fully crusted.

HARDCORE

Reye's syndrome (acute encephalopathy) is a feared complication that may develop in children with a varicella infection concurrently ingesting salicylates (aspirin). Reye's has a mortality rate of 10% to 40%, and despite the link with varicella and concomitant aspirin ingestion, the pathogenesis is unknown.

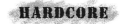

HARDCORE

Infants infected by *C. botulinum* become ill following the ingestion of *C. botulinum* spores, which grow within the infants intestines and release toxins. Adults may also become infected by *C. botulinum;* however, adult botulism occurs after a person eats food that contains the preformed botulism toxin, not necessarily the spores. This typically occurs due to improper food canning and/or refrigeration.

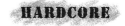

HARDCORE

Clostridia are ancient organisms that live in anaerobic habitats (soils, aquatic sediments, and the intestinal tracts of animals).

HARDCORE

Without treatment, adult *Enterobius* females can live for approximately 3 months.

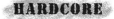

HARDCORE

Adenovirus cells may have small eosinophilic or basophilic inclusions that can enlarge and obscure the nuclear membrane. The cells are referred to as **"smudge" cells**.

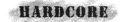

V. DERMATOLOGICAL

A. Bacteria

Streptococcus pyogenes
- Gram-positive cocci in chains
- Catalase –
- Group A Lancefield
- Facultative anaerobe

CLINICAL CORRELATES—IMPETIGO
➤ Impetigo is a local skin infection caused by normal skin flora (mostly *S. pyogenes*, but also *S. aureus*) that consists of superficial blisters whose surface is covered with pus or crust that appears as *"honey-colored" crusting*. Impetigo occurs most commonly at the angle of the mouth, around nasal flares, and behind the ears.

➤ Facial impetigo can be dangerous if it spreads to the cavernous sinus.

B. Viruses

Human Papillomavirus (HPV)
- Double-stranded, circular DNA virus
- Papovaviridae

CLINICAL CORRELATES—VERRUCA VULGARIS (COMMON WARTS)
➤ Common warts are well-demarcated, rough, hard nodules typically found on hands. This infection is typically asymptomatic but cosmetically not very attractive, and can also be removed with curettage, cryotherapy, or laser therapies.

Molluscum contagiosum
- Double-stranded, DNA virus
- Poxvirus

CLINICAL CORRELATES—WARTS
➤ *Molluscum* is a poxvirus that replicates in the cytoplasm of host cells. This virus causes a localized infection characterized by *dome-shaped papules* with a shiny surface and central indentation or **umbilication**. The lesions may appear anywhere on the body *except the palms and soles* and are spread by direct skin-to-skin contact.

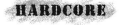

Although these infections are self-limited and spontaneously resolve after a few months, *M. contagiosum* warts can be removed with curettage, cryotherapy, or laser therapies.

C. Fungi

Tinea
- Dermatophyte

CLINICAL CORRELATES—RINGWORM (TINEA CAPITIS, TINEA CORPORIS), JOCK ITCH (TINEA CRURIS), ATHLETE'S FOOT (TINEA PEDIS), AND ONYCHOMYCOSIS (TINEA UNGUIUM)
➤ Tinea capitis, *ringworm of the scalp*, occurs almost always in small children.

➤ Tinea pedis, ringworm of the feet (**athlete's foot**), is the most common dermatophyte infection.

➤ Tinea unguium, ringworm of the nails, is also known as **dermatophytic onychomycosis**.

➤ Tinea corporis is ringworm of *glabrous skin* (skin normally devoid of hair).

➤ Tinea cruris (**jock itch**) is a special form of tinea corporis involving the crural fold.

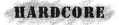

Diagnosis of tinea infection should be confirmed by **KOH examination** of scrapings from the lesions.

VI. OPTHALMOLOGICAL

Conjunctivitis means "inflammation of the conjunctiva" and is commonly encountered in children with red eyes and watery or purulent discharge.

A. Bacterial

- *Streptococcus pneumoniae*
- *Haemophilus influenzae*
- *Moraxella catarrhalis*

Bacterial conjunctivitis is spread by direct contact of secretions and is highly contagious. Bacterial conjunctivitis typically **begins in one eye** and consists of redness, irritation, and **purulent discharge** that continues throughout the day.

Chlamydia trachomatis

- Gram-negative
- Obligate intracellular parasite

CLINICAL CORRELATES—NEONATAL CONJUNCTIVITIS

➤ Chlamydial infection is the **most common cause of conjunctivitis in the neonatal period**. Infection follows passage through an infected birth canal and presents with **purulent eye discharge**, marked swelling of the eyelids, and eventually a **pseudomembrane** that forms as the exudate adheres to the conjunctiva.

B. Viral

Adenovirus

- Double-stranded DNA
- Naked virus
- Icosahedral nucleocapsid

CLINICAL CORRELATES—VIRAL CONJUNCTIVITIS

➤ **Viral conjunctivitis is most commonly caused by adenovirus**. Adenovirus conjunctivitis is highly contagious and spread by direct contact. Viral conjunctivitis presents as redness, **watery or mucoserous discharge**, and a burning sensation that typically **begins in both eyes** (remember, bacterial conjunctivitis begins in one eye) after autoinoculation following primary infection in one eye.

VII. EAR INFECTIONS

A. Otitis Media

- *Streptococcus pneumoniae*
- *Haemophilus influenzae*
- *Moraxella catarrhalis*

Otitis media is an infection of the middle ear that most commonly occurs in children between 6 and 24 months of age. Typical clinical symptoms include ear pain, hearing loss, and vertigo.

B. Otitis Externa

- *Pseudomonas aeruginosa*
- *Staphylococcus aureus*

External otitis is inflammation of the external auditory canal and is most commonly caused by *P. aeruginosa*. This infection is commonly referred to as "swimmer's ear" because people involved with water activities are at a greater risk for *P. aeruginosa* exposure.

VIII. MUSCULOSKELETAL

A. Bacteria

Pseudomonas aeruginosa

- Gram-negative rod
- Aerobe
- Oxidase +
- Non-lactose fermenter

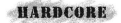

If untreated, *Chlamydia* conjunctival infection can cause corneal and conjunctival scarring, leading to blindness.

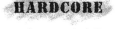

S. pneumoniae is the most common bacterial cause of otitis media.

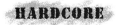

Patients with otitis externa will have pain in the external ear when the pinnea is tugged. In otitis media, pain is only in the internal ear and these patients will not react to external ear manipulation.

CLINICAL CORRELATES—OSTEOMYELITIS

➤ Classically, a child develops *P. aeruginosa* osteomyelitis of the foot after stepping on a *rusty nail that punctures their foot through a tennis shoe*.

HARDCORE REVIEW TABLES–INFECTIONS IN NEONATES, INFANTS, AND CHILDREN (TABLE 2-2 TO TABLE 2-9)

TABLE 2-2	The Most Common Organisms That Cause Meningitis		
	#1 Bug	**#2 Bug**	**#3 Bug**
Newborns	Group B *Streptococcus*	*Listeria monocytogenes*	*Streptococcus pneumoniae*
1 month to 2 years	*Streptococcus pneumoniae*	*Neisseria meningitidis*	Group B *Streptococcus*
2 to 18 years	*Neisseria meningitidis*	*Streptococcus pneumoniae*	*Haemophilus influenzae*

TABLE 2-3	Rash Recognition in Children	
Infection	**Etiology**	**Rash Characteristics**
Chickenpox	Varicella-zoster virus	• Crops of papules that become vesicles • Erythematous base • Marked pruritis
Gingivostomatitis	Herpes simplex virus 1/2	• Halitosis • Friable mucosa • Fever
Roseola	HHV-6, HHV-7	• Exanthem subitum • Onset within 24 hours of fever • Central distribution • Patient less toxic appearing than expected
Scarlet fever	Group A beta-hemolytic streptococci	• Onset in 24 hours • Appears like a "sunburn with goosebumps" • Sandpaper feel • Petechial accentuation in skin folds • Facial flush with circumoral pallor
Shingles	Varicella-zoster virus	• Pain before rash • Groups of small vesicles in dermatomal distribution

TABLE 2-4	Central Nervous System		
Bugs	**Bug Points**	**Most Common Presentation**	**Hardcore Microbiology**
Gram-Positive Bacteria			
Listeria monocytogenes	• Facultative-intracellular gram-positive bacillus • Catalase + • Facultative anaerobe	Newborn meningitis	Transmission via ingestion of contaminated raw milk or cheese
Streptococcus agalactiae: Group B Streptococcus (GBS)	• Gram-positive coccus in chains • Group B, beta-hemolytic • Facultative anaerobe	Neonatal meningitis	Part of normal vaginal flora (30–40% of pregnant women)
Streptococcus pneumoniae	• Gram-positive, lancet-shaped *Diplococcus* in chains • Catalase – • Ferments inulin Optochin-sensitive (+ Quellung reaction) • Alpha-hemolytic	Meningitis in children (1 month to 2 years) and adults, conjunctivitis	Alpha-hemolysis on blood agar, part of normal oropharyngeal flora

(Continued)

TABLE 2-4	Central Nervous System (Cont.)		
BUGS	**BUG POINTS**	**MOST COMMON PRESENTATION**	**HARDCORE MICROBIOLOGY**
Gram-Negative Bacteria			
Haemophilus influenzae	• Gram-negative rod • Oxidase + • Non-lactose fermenter • Aerobe	Meningitis in kids 2–18 years of age	Children are immunized with the Hib vaccine, which contains type b capsular polysacular polysaccharide conjugated to diphtheria toxoid, is not airborne
Neisseria meningitidis	• Gram-negative diplococci • Ferments maltose and glucose • Oxidase + • Anaerobe	Meningitis in children and young adults	Kidney bean shape, high risk for newborns (>1 month of age) and army recruits, look for accompanying petechial rash

TABLE 2-5	Pulmonary		
BUGS	**BUG POINTS**	**MOST COMMON PRESENTATION**	**HARDCORE MICROBIOLOGY**
Gram-Positive Bacteria			
Corynebacterium diphtheriae	• Gram-positive rod • Catalase + • Anaerobe • Non-spore forming	Pseudomembranous pharyngitis	Treat with DPT (diptheria, pertussis, tetanus) vaccination, penicillin, and antitoxin Diptheria toxin (beta-prophage) inhibits the translation of human mRNA by inhibiting EF-2 via ADP ribosylation
Streptococcus agalactiae: Group B *Streptococcus* (GBS)	• Gram-positive coccus in chains • Group B, beta-hemolytic • Facultative anaerobe	Neonatal pneumonia	Part of normal vaginal flora (30-40% of pregnant women)
Streptococcus pneumoniae	• Gram-positive coccus in chains • Catalase − • Ferments inulin • Optochin sensitive (+ Quellung reaction) • Alpha-hemolytic	Community-acquired pneumonia	Alpha-hemolysis on blood agar, part of normal or opharyngeal flora
Streptococcus pyogenes	• Gram-positive cocci in chains • Catalase − • Group A Lancefield • Facultative anaerobe	Bacterial pharyngitis or "Strep throat," scarlet fever, rheumatic fever, poststreptococcal glomerulonephritis, impetigo	Produces erythrogenic exotoxins, beta-hemolytic
Gram-Negative Bacteria			
Bordetella pertussis	• Gram-negative coccobacillus • Aerobic	Whooping cough	Three stages of disease, cultured on Regan-Lowe medium
Chlamydia trachomatis	• Gram-negative • Obligate intracellular parasite	Pneumonia	Subtypes L1, L2, L3
Mycoplasma			
Mycoplasma pneumoniae	• Pleomorphic • No cell wall	Community-acquired pneumonia (atypical)	Diagnosed with cold agglutinins, CXR appears worse than clinical picture
Viruses			
Adenovirus	• Double-stranded DNA • Naked virus • Icosahedral nucleocapsid	Upper respiratory tract infection	Prevalent in daycare centers
Human herpesvirus 6	• Double-stranded, DNA virus • Gamma herpesvirus • Icosahedral nucleocapsid	Roseola infantum	Latent infection of the T lymphocyte, look for morbilliform rash following high fever
Influenza A and B virus	• Negative, single-stranded, RNA virus • Orthomyxovirus	Pneumonia	Associated with Guillain-Barré syndrome and Reye's syndrome
Parainfluenza virus	• Single-stranded RNA virus • *Parmyxoviridae*	Croup	Hallmark of a croup infection is a barking cough

(Continued)

TABLE 2-5 Pulmonary (Cont.)

BUGS	BUG POINTS	MOST COMMON PRESENTATION	HARDCORE MICROBIOLOGY
Parvovirus B 19	• Single-stranded, DNA virus • *Parvoviridae* • Icosahedral nucleocapsid	Erythema infectiosum (fifth disease)	The smallest DNA virus
Respiratory syncytial virus	• Negative, single-stranded RNA virus • Paramyxovirus	Upper and lower respiratory tract infection	Produces syncytial effect of cell fusion in infected cells, very common in kids <1 year old

TABLE 2-6 Other Important Pediatric Viral Infections

BUGS	BUG POINTS	MOST COMMON PRESENTATION	HARDCORE MICROBIOLOGY
Measles virus	• Negative, single-stranded RNA virus • *Paramyxovirus*	Measles (rubeola)	Koplik's spots on buccal mucosa, maculopapular rash with cranial-to-caudal progression
Mumps virus	• Negative, single-stranded RNA virus • *Paramyxovirus*	Mumps	Complications include orchitis and parotitis
Varicella-zoster virus (human herpesvirus 3)	• Double-stranded, DNA virus • Herpesvirus alpha • Icosahedral nucleocapsid	Chickenpox	Diagnose with Tzanck smear or fluorescent antibody staining

TABLE 2-7 Gastrointestinal

BUGS	BUG POINTS	MOST COMMON PRESENTATION	HARDCORE MICROBIOLOGY
Gram-Positive Bacteria			
Clostridium botulinum	• Gram-positive rod • Anaerobe • Endospores	Botulism	"Floppy baby" appearance after ingesting honey
Parasites			
Enterobius vermicularis	• Helminth • Intestinal nematode	Pinworm infestation	Fecal–oral transmission with perianal itching, diagnosed with Scotch-tape test
Viruses			
Adenovirus	• Double-stranded DNA • Naked virus • Icosahedral nucleocapsid	Diarrhea	Asymmetrical replication in the nucleus of epithelial cells, prevalent in daycare centers
Rotavirus	• Double-stranded, DNA virus • Reovirus	Diarrhea	Replicates in cytoplasm

TABLE 2-8 Dermatology

BUGS	BUG POINTS	MOST COMMON PRESENTATION	HARDCORE MICROBIOLOGY
Gram-Positive Bacteria			
Streptococcus pyogenes	• Gram-positive cocci in chains • Catalase – • Group A Lancefield • Facultative anaerobe	Impetigo	Appears as "honey-colored" crusting
Viruses			
Human papillomavirus	• Double-stranded, circular DNA virus • Papovaviridae	Verruca vulgaris (common warts)	Typically found on hands
Molluscum contagiosum	• Double-stranded, DNA virus • Poxvirus	Warts	Characterized by dome-shaped papules with a shiny surface and central indentation or umbilication
Fungi			
Tinea • Capitis • Corporis • Cruris • Pedis • Unguium	Dermatophyte	Ringworm (tinea corporis), ringworm of the scalp (tinea capitis), jock itch (tinea cruris), athlete's foot (tinea pedis), and onychomycosis (tinea unguium)	Tinea infection confirmed with KOH prep

TABLE 2-9	Musculoskeletal		
Bugs	**Bug Points**	**Most Common Presentation**	**Hardcore Microbiology**
Gram-Negative Bacteria			
Pseudomonas aeruginosa	• Gram-negative rod • Aerobe • Oxidase + • Non-lactose fermenter	Osteomyelitis	Develops after stepping on a rusty nail that punctures a child's foot through their tennis shoe

CHAPTER 3

Infections of Pregnant Women

Congenital infections are acquired *in utero*, or during passage of the neonate through the birth canal, and are an important cause of fetal and neonatal morbidity and mortality. The most important congenital infections can be remembered with the acronym "*TORCH*":

- Toxoplasmosis
- Other (syphilis)
- Rubella
- Cytomegalovirus (CMV)
- Herpes simplex virus (HSV)

All pregnant mothers receiving prenatal care and newborns should be routinely screened for these infections.

Bugs discussed in this chapter:

- *Toxoplasma gondii*
- *Treponema pallidum*
- *Rubivirus*

- *Cytomegalovirus*
- Herpes simplex virus
- Hepatitis E

Toxoplasma gondii

- Protozoa
- Obligate intracellular parasite
- Trophozoites
- Oocyst

CLINICAL CORRELATES—CONGENITAL TOXOPLASMOSIS

➤ *T. gondii* is a protozoa that uses cats as a host and is transmitted to humans via *cat feces*. If a pregnant woman is exposed to *T. gondii*, congenital toxoplasmosis infection may result, manifesting as neonate *chorioretinitis, hydrocephalus, and intracranial calcifications*.

➤ In adult human infections, *Toxoplasma* trophozoites form *cysts* in muscle and brain tissue.

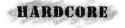

Remember that *T. gondii* is acquired primarily from the intake of undercooked or raw meat, especially in underdeveloped countries.

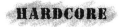

Just as toxoplasmosis causes *intracranial* cysts in infected adults, it causes *intracranial* calcifications in neonates.

Treponema pallidum

- Gram-negative, corkscrew shaped
- Spirochete

CLINICAL CORRELATES—CONGENITAL SYPHILIS

➤ Neonatal syphilis is acquired by direct infant contact with maternal ulcerative lesions, or via transplacental transmission. This infection can result in fetal stillbirth, hydrops fetalis, frontal bossing, short maxilla, high palatal arch, or the **Hutchinson triad**: Hutchinson teeth (blunted upper incisors), interstitial keratitis, and eighth-nerve deafness.

➤ Screening for congenital syphilis involves nontreponemal testing, either *VDRL or RPR*. If the resulting screening test is positive, diagnosis should be confirmed with specific treponemal serologic testing (fluorescent treponemal antibody absorption *[FTA-ABS]*).

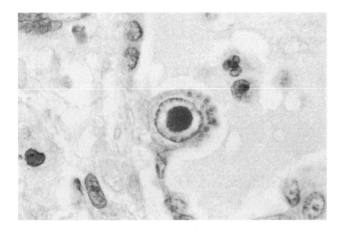

Figure 3-1 Lung tissue with characteristic "owl's-eye." Cytomegalovirus nuclear inclusion and cytoplasmic inclusions. *Reprinted with permission from McClatchey KD. Clinical Laboratory Medicine, 2nd Edition. Philadelphia: Lippincott Williams & Wilkins, 2002.*

Rubivirus

- Positive, single-stranded RNA virus
- *Togaviridae*
- Nonsegmented

CLINICAL CORRELATES—CONGENITAL RUBELLA SYNDROME

➤ Congenital rubella may cause neonatal deafness, cataracts, patent ductus arteriosus, neurologic sequelae, thrombocytopenia, or purpuric skin lesions classically described as **"blueberry muffin" lesions**.

Cytomegalovirus

- Double-stranded DNA
- Herpesvirus
- Icosahedral nucleocapsid

CLINICAL CORRELATES—CONGENITAL CYTOMEGALOVIRAL INFECTION

➤ Congenital CMV is the *most common congenital viral infection*. This infection occurs via *transplacental transmission* of the virus following primary maternal infection or reactivation of a latent virus.

➤ Infants suffering from congenital CMV infection may present with jaundice, enlarged liver, petechial rash, microcephaly, chorioretinitis, or cerebral calcifications.

- To remember congenital **CMV** infection:
  - **C**horioretinitis
  - **M**icrocephally
  - li**V**er dysfunction—jaundice, hepatomegaly

Herpes Simplex Virus

- Double-stranded, linear DNA virus
- *Herpesviridae*

CLINICAL CORRELATES—CONGENITAL HERPES SIMPLEX VIRAL INFECTION

➤ HSV is primarily transmitted to an infant through an *infected maternal genital tract*, although intrauterine infection may also occur.

➤ Clinical manifestations occur in three patterns: *localization to the skin*, eyes, or mouth; *CNS disease*; or *disseminated disease* to multiple organs leading to hypotension, jaundice, DIC, apnea, and shock.

Hepatitis E

- Positive, linear, single-stranded RNA virus
- *Calicivirus*

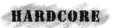

Congenital rubella is classically described as a "blueberry muffin baby" with cataracts.

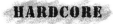

CMV is diagnosed by finding *intranuclear inclusion bodies* surrounded by halos, referred to as **"owl's eyes"** (Fig. 3-1).

CLINICAL CORRELATES—WATER-BORNE NEONATAL HEPATITIS

➤ Hepatitis E is an enterically transmitted water-borne hepatitis that most commonly occurs in developing countries. This form of hepatitis can be very serious in pregnant women, potentially resulting in fatal complications.

• Remember that hepatitis "E" occurs in Expectant mothers.

TABLE 3-1	TORCH (with Hepatitis E)		
BUGS	**BUG POINTS**	**MOST COMMON PRESENTATION**	**HARDCORE MICROBIOLOGY**
Toxoplasma gondii			
	• Protozoa • Obligate intracellular parasite • Trophozoites • Oocyst	Congenital toxoplasmosis ○ Chorioretinitis ○ Hydrocephalus ○ Intracranial calcifications	Transmission occurs via cat feces
Treponema pallidum			

	• Gram-negative,
	  corkscrew shaped
	• Spirochete
		Congenital syphilis
		○ Fetal stillbirth
		○ Hydrops fetalis
		○ Frontal bossing
		○ Short maxilla
		○ High palatal arch
		  Hutchinson triad:
		  Hutchinson teeth
		  (blunted upper incisors),
		  interstitial keratitis,
		  eighth-nerve deafness
			Screen mandatory in pregnant women using nontreponemal testing (VDRL or RPR), if positive diagnosis is confirmed with specific treponemal serologic testing (fluorescent treponemal antibody absorption (FTA-ABS)

Rubivirus			
	• Positive, single-stranded RNA virus • *Togaviridae* • Nonsegmented	Congenital rubella syndrome ○ Neonatal deafness ○ Cataracts ○ Patent ductus arteriosus ○ Neurologic sequelae ○ Thrombocytopenia ○ Purpuric skin lesion	Classically a "blueberry muffin baby" with cataracts
Cytomegalovirus			
	• Double-stranded DNA • Herpes virus • Icosahedral nucleocapsid	Congenital cytomegalo viral infection ○ Jaundice ○ Enlarged liver ○ Petechial rash ○ Microcephaly ○ Chorioretinitis ○ Cerebral calcifications	Most common congenital viral infection
Herpes Simplex Virus			
	• Double-stranded, linear DNA virus • *Herpesviridae*	Congenital herpes simplex viral infection ○ Hypotension ○ Jaundice ○ DIC ○ Apnea ○ Shock	Transmitted to an infant through an infected maternal genital tract
Hepatitis E			
	• Positive, linear, single- stranded RNA virus • *Calicivirus*	Water-borne neonatal hepatitis	Occurs in pregnant women in developing countries

CHAPTER 4

Infections Associated with a Rash on the Hands and Feet

Although rashes are a common and typically nondescript symptom associated with many illnesses, a rash that includes the hands and feet is characteristically seen only in a small subset of infections. Therefore, it is important for you to remember these bugs, which characteristically cause a rash of the hands and feet.

Bugs discussed in this chapter:

- Coxsackievirus
- *Rickettsia* organism
- *Treponema pallidum*

A. Gram-Negative Bacteria

Rickettsia ricketsii

- Gram-negative
- Obligate intracellular bacterium

CLINICAL CORRELATES—ROCKY MOUNTAIN SPOTTED FEVER

➤ Rocky Mountain spotted fever is caused by *Rickettsia rickettsii* and spread by a tick vector. Symptoms include fever, hepatosplenomegaly, and rash that first appears on the extremities, including the palms and soles of the feet, and then moves to the body.

➤ *Rickettsia* organisms are harbored by a variety of arthropods including **ticks, mites, and the human louse**.

➤ *Rickettsia* may require **Giemsa stain** for visualization.

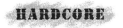

HARDCORE

The rash of RMSF spreads in the opposite direction of the rash of Lyme disease, which first starts on the body and moves to the extremities.

Treponema pallidum

- Gram-negative, corkscrew shaped
- Spirochete

CLINICAL CORRELATES—SECONDARY SYPHILIS INFECTION

➤ A red maculopapular rash that extends over the entire body, including the hands and feet, is characteristic of a **secondary syphilis infection**. Typically, secondary syphilis infection appears within 2 to 10 weeks following an untreated primary syphilis infection and occurs with condylomata lata (pale papules in the anogenital region).

➤ *T. pallidum* is visualized with **darkfield microscopy**.

B. Viruses

Coxsackievirus

- Single-stranded, linear RNA virus
- Picornavirus

CLINICAL CORRELATES—HAND-FOOT-AND-MOUTH DISEASE

➤ Hand-foot-and-mouth disease, caused by **coxsackie virus A**, is characterized by oral and pharyngeal ulcerations along with a **vesicular rash of the palms and soles of the feet**. This illness is

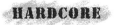

HARDCORE

These enteroviruses are divided into two groups, **coxsackie A and B**:

- *Coxsackie A*—**Hand-foot-and-mouth disease**, acute conjunctivitis.
- *Coxsackie B*—Pleurodynia, myocarditis, pericarditis, encephalitis.

common in the spring and is spread by vesicular contact, pharyngeal secretions, and fecal–oral contact. Symptomatic treatment only.

• Remember: Coxsackie **B** infections are generally more severe than A, thus remember that "**B** is **B**ad."

HARDCORE REVIEW TABLE—INFECTIONS ASSOCIATED WITH A RASH ON THE HANDS AND FEET (TABLE 4-1)

TABLE 4-1	Rash on the Hands and Feet		
BUGS	**BUG POINTS**	**MOST COMMON PRESENTATION**	**HARDCORE MICROBIOLOGY**
Gram-Negative Bacteria			
Rickettsia ricketsii	• Gram-negative • Obligate intracellular • Obligate intracellular bacterium	• Rocky Mountain spotted fever (*Rickettsia ricketsii*)	Spread by ticks, mites, and human louse, Giemsa stain
Treponema pallidum	• Gram-negative, corkscrew shaped • Spirochete	Syphilis—secondary	Condylomata lata also seen during secondary syphilis infection, diagnosis with darkfield microscopy
Coxsackievirus	• Single-stranded, linear RNA virus • Picornavirus	Hand-foot-and-mouth disease	Two subtypes include coxsackie A and B (A associated with hand-and-foot rash)

CHAPTER 5

Infections of Healthy Adults and the Elderly

The following bugs are common offenders for causing infection in normal healthy adults, especially among the elderly population.

Bugs discussed in this chapter:

- *Streptococcus pneumoniae*
- *Neisseria meningitidis*
- *Enterovirus*
- Herpes simplex virus
- *Staphylococcus saprophyticus*
- *Escherichia coli*
- *Candida albicans*

- *Staphylococcus aureus*
- *Streptococcus pyogenes*
- *Chlamydia pneumoniae*
- *Rhinovirus*
- *Pseudomonas aeruginosa*
- Varicella-zoster virus
- Human herpesvirus 7

I. CENTRAL NERVOUS SYSTEM

Meningitis is a serious illness that is most commonly encountered in the pediatric population; however, adults can also develop CNS infections. Be aware of the following bugs in any adult or elderly patient who presents with headache and nuchal rigidity. Remember that the diagnosis of meningitis requires analysis of cerebral spinal fluid (CSF) via lumbar puncture for culture and cytology.

A. Gram-Positive Bacteria

Streptococcus pneumoniae

- Gram-positive, lancet-shaped diplococcus in chains
- Catalase –
- Ferments inulin
- Optochin-sensitive
- Alpha-hemolytic
- Facultative anaerobe

CLINICAL CORRELATES—BACTERIA MENINGITIS

➤ *S. pneumoniae* is the **most common cause of meningitis in both healthy adults and the elderly**. Any finding of gram-positive diplococci in the CSF is most likely pneumococcal infection.

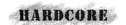

HARDCORE

CSF findings suggestive of bacterial meningitis include a **low glucose** concentration (<45 mg/dL) **high protein** concentration (>500 mg/dL) and a **white cell count** above 1,000/μL.

B. Gram-Negative Bacteria

Neisseria meningitidis

- Gram-negative diplococci
- Ferments maltose and glucose
- Oxidase +
- Anaerobe

CLINICAL CORRELATES—MENINGITIS IN YOUNG ADULTS, ESPECIALLY BREAKOUTS ON COLLEGE CAMPUSES AND IN MILITARY BOOT CAMPS

➤ *N. meningitidis* is the second most common cause of adult bacterial meningitis behind *S. pneumoniae*. Diagnose *N. meningitides* with **positive CSF oxidase test and cultures**.

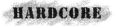

HARDCORE

In a patient with meningeal signs and a petechial rash, think of meningococcal meningitis.

C. Viruses

Enterovirus

- Positive, single-stranded RNA virus
- *Picornaviridae*
- Nonsegmented

CLINICAL CORRELATES—ASEPTIC MENINGITIS (NONBACTERIAL MENINGITIS), ENCEPHALITIS

➤ Enteroviruses are responsible for up to 70% of adult viral meningitis and encephalitis. Aseptic meningitis presents with a fever up to 40°C, headache, meningismus, nausea, and vomiting.

➤ Transmission of enteroviruses occurs mainly via the *fecal–oral* route, but also through contact with infected respiratory secretions.

Herpes Simplex Virus

- Double-stranded, linear DNA virus
- *Herpesviridae*

CLINICAL CORRELATES—ASEPTIC MENINIGITIS, ENCEPHALITIS

➤ Herpes simplex virus consists of two serotypes, HSV-1 and HSV-2. **HSV-1** is typically responsible for oral ulcers and encephalitis, while **HSV-2** is associated with genital lesions and meningitis.

II. GENITOURINARY SYSTEM

A. Gram-Positive Bacteria

Staphylococcus saprophyticus

- Gram-positive cocci in clusters
- Coagulase –
- Catalase +
- Facultative anaerobe

CLINICAL CORRELATES—ACUTE CYSTITIS (BLADDER INFECTION)

➤ *Staphylococcus saprophyticus* is a common cause of *cystitis in young women*. Although *E. coli* is responsible for a majority of acute cystitis cases, *S. saprophyticus* accounts for most other episodes.

➤ This organism is able to infect the bladder by using a *lactosamine residue* that allows it to strongly adhere to the bladder urothelium.

B. Gram-Negative Bacteria

Escherichia coli

- Gram-negative rod
- Beta-hemolytic
- Lactose fermenter
- Indole +
- Facultative anaerobe

CLINICAL CORRELATES—URINARY TRACT INFECTION, ACUTE CYSTITIS

➤ *E. coli* is the causative pathogen in most episodes of cystitis, which present with dysuria, frequency, urgency, and suprapubic pain.

C. Fungi

Candida albicans

- Pseudohyphae and true hyphae
- Oval-budding yeast

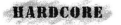

Diagnosis of HSV meningitis is made by positive CSF viral cultures and the detection of HSV DNA by PCR, or with *Tzanck smear* (HSV-1) when skin lesions are involved.

HARDCORE

Genital lesions may also be present in patients with HSV-2 meningitis.

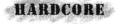

In the elderly, urinary tract infections can cause altered mental status resembling delirium and dementia.

CLINICAL CORRELATES–VULVOVAGINAL CANDIDIASIS

➤ *C. albicans* is the **most common cause of vulvovaginal candidiasis**. Patients with vulvovaginal candidiasis will complain of vulvar puritis, dysuria, and a **white, clumpy, curd-like discharge**. Several factors may predispose women to *Candida* infection including:

1. Antibiotics, which inhibit normal vaginal bacterial flora.

2. Use of oral contraceptives that contain high levels of estrogen.

3. Contraceptive devices.

4. Pregnancy.

5. Immunosuppression, including corticosteroid use and HIV infection.

III. MUSCULOSKELETAL SYSTEM

Osteomyelitis is a bone infection that results in inflammatory bone destruction and formation of new bone. Osteomyelitis can develop through three mechanisms of infection:

1. Osteomyelitis secondary to direct inoculation (e.g., after trauma, surgery, or insertion of a prosthetic joint).

2. Osteomyelitis in patients with chronic vascular insufficiency, primarily occurring in patients with diabetes mellitus and/or peripheral vascular disease.

3. Osteomyelitis following hematogenous spread of infection.

Acute osteomyelitis can evolve over several weeks to chronic osteomyelitis, which is associated with the presence of dead bone, reactive bony encasement of the dead bone, local bone loss, and the development of sinus tracts (extensions through cortical bone that drain through the skin).

Staphylococcus aureus

- Gram-positive cocci (clusters)
- Catalase +
- Coagulase +
- Beta-hemolytic

CLINICAL CORRELATES—OSTEOMYELITIS

➤ *S. aureus* is the primary organism that causes osteomyelitis in the adult population. *S. aureus* infects bone by hematological seeding or via direct inoculation. *S. aureus* is able to adhere to bone matrix components via the expression of specific **adhesins**. The organism also possesses fibronectin-binding proteins that coat foreign bodies, and are particularly important in **infections associated with prosthetic joints**.

➤ *S. aureus* secretes two main toxins, **exotoxin and toxic shock syndrome toxin (TSST-1)**, both of which suppress plasma cell differentiation, stimulate production of cytokines, and subvert the cellular and humoral immune system. Primary exotoxins produced by *S. aureus* include lipases (hydrolyzes lipids), leukocidin (lyse WBCs), exfoilatin (lyse epithelial cells), staphylokinase (activates plasminogen), and penicillinase (destroys penicillins).

IV. PULMONARY SYSTEM

A. Gram-Positive Bacteria

Streptococcus pneumoniae

- Gram-positive, lancet-shaped diplococcus in chains
- Catalase –
- Ferments inulin
- Optochin-sensitive
- Alpha-hemolytic
- Facultative anaerobe

CLINICAL CORRELATES—COMMUNITY-ACQUIRED, LOBAR PNEUMONIA

➤ *S. pneumoniae* is the **most common cause of community-acquired pneumonia**. This organism typically localizes to a single lung lobe and therefore is referred to as **lobar bacterial pneumonia**. Lobar pneumonia is easily identified on chest X-ray by a dense consolidation in the lung.

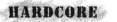

HARDCORE

Vulvovaginal candidiasis is not considered a sexually transmitted disease.

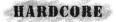

HARDCORE

Vulvovaginal candidiasis is diagnosed by **KOH preparation**, which reveals the characteristic branching yeast and hyphae.

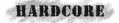

HARDCORE

Hematogenously spread *S. aureus* osteomyelitis most commonly occurs in the vertebral column.

➤ *S. pneumoniae* is part of the normal oropharyngeal flora, but can cause infection after localizing to the alveolus. *S. pneumoniae* initially invades the alveolar epithelium and passes from alveolus to alveolus, creating inflammation and consolidation along lobar compartments.

B. Gram-Negative Bacteria

Chlamydia pneumoniae
- Gram-negative
- Obligate intracellular parasite

CLINICAL CORRELATES—LOWER RESPIRATORY TRACT INFECTION, PNEUMONIA

➤ *C. pneumoniae* causes a nonspecific pneumonia with higher incidence in the elderly. Diagnosis is made with PCR or by the detection of antibodies or antigens in nasopharyngeal swabs.

C. Viruses

Rhinovirus
- Single-stranded, RNA virus
- *Picornaviridae*

CLINICAL CORRELATES—COMMON COLD

➤ Rhinoviruses are associated with the common cold. These viruses are spread when infected nasal secretions *enter the nasopharynx through the nasal or ophthalmic mucosa* (e.g., picking your nose or rubbing your eyes after contact with infected secretions).

➤ Treatment is symptomatic.

- Remember—"rhino" means "nose"!

V. DERMATOLOGICAL SYSTEM

A. Gram-Positive Bacteria

Staphylococcus aureus
- Gram-positive cocci (clusters)
- Catalase +
- Coagulase +
- Beta-hemolytic

CLINICAL CORRELATES—FURUNCLE, CELLULITIS

➤ *S. aureus* is the most common cause of **furunculosis**, a painful nodular lesion that drains pus. These develop when hair follicles are exposed to friction and perspiration, commonly occurring in people who are obese, on corticosteroid therapy, or have deficient neutrophil function.

➤ *S. aureus*, along with *S. pyogenes*, is the main bug responsible for cellulitis.

Streptococcus pyogenes
- Gram-positive cocci in chains
- Catalase –
- Group A Lancefield
- Facultative anaerobe

CLINICAL CORRELATES—CELLULITIS, ERYSIPELAS

➤ Cellulitis is an acute and spreading infection of the skin and subcutaneous tissues. Typically, it occurs when organisms of the normal skin flora gain access to the subcutaneous layer via a small break in the skin from wounds, burns, or surgical incisions.

➤ If the lesion spreads from the subcutaneous layer, it may cause massive edema and a rapidly advancing margin of infection, which is called *erysipelas*.

B. Gram-Negative Bacteria

Pseudomonas aeruginosa

- Gram-negative rod
- Aerobe
- Oxidase +
- Nonlactose fermenter

CLINICAL CORRELATES—"HOT TUB" FOLLICULITIS

➤ Folliculitis is a superficial bacterial infection of hair follicles characterized by small, white-headed pimples. Exposure to whirlpools, swimming pools, and hot tubs contaminated with *Pseudomonas aeruginosa* and with inadequate chlorination can result in **"hot tub" folliculitis**.

C. Viruses

Human Herpesvirus 7

- Linear, double-stranded DNA virus

CLINICAL CORRELATES—PITYRIASIS ROSEA

➤ HHV-7 is a lymphotropic virus that replicates in CD4+ T lymphocytes and results in pityriasis rosea in young adults. Pityriasis infection begins as a *salmon-colored, "herald" patch lesion* on the chest, neck, or back. The lesion becomes scaly and other lesions develop along lines of skin cleavage in what is known as a **"Christmas tree" distribution**.

➤ The rash resolves spontaneously.

Varicella-Zoster Virus

- Double-stranded, DNA virus
- Herpesvirus alpha
- Icosahedral nucleocapsid

CLINICAL CORRELATES—HERPES-ZOSTER ("SHINGLES")

➤ Herpes-zoster, or "shingles," occurs when a *latent varicella-zoster infection within sensory ganglia is reactivated*. This illness is characterized by a painful, unilateral vesicular eruption localized in a *dermatomal distribution*.

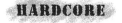

HARDCORE REVIEW TABLES—INFECTIONS OF HEALTHY ADULTS AND THE ELDERLY (TABLE 5-1 TO TABLE 5-5)

HARDCORE

VZV can be diagnosed with *Tzanck smear* or fluorescent antibody staining.

TABLE 5-1	Central Nervous System		
BUGS	**BUG POINTS**	**MOST COMMON PRESENTATION**	**HARDCORE MICROBIOLOGY**
Gram-Positive Bacteria			
Streptococcus pneumoniae	• Gram-positive, lancet-shaped diplococcus in chains • Catalase – • Ferments inulin • Optochin-sensitive • Alpha-hemolytic • Facultative anaerobe	Bacterial meningitis	Most common cause of meningitis in both healthy adults and the elderly
Gram-Negative Bacteria			
Neisseria meningitidis	• Gram-negative diplococci • Ferments maltose and glucose • Oxidase + • Anaerobe	Meningitis in young adults	Breakouts on college campuses and military boot camps, petechial rash
Viruses			
Enterovirus	• Positive, single-stranded RNA virus • Picornaviridae • Nonsegmented	Aseptic meningitis, encephalitis	Fever up to 40°C, transmission via fecal–oral route (most common), and contact with infected respiratory secretions
Herpes Simplex Virus	• Double-stranded, linear DNA virus • *Herpesviridae*	Aseptic meningitis, encephalitis	Two serotypes—HSV 1 and 2: ○ HSV-1 is responsible for oral ulcers and encephalitis, while ○ HSV-2 is associated with genital lesions and meningitis

TABLE 5-2	Genitourinary System		
BUGS	**BUG POINTS**	**MOST COMMON PRESENTATION**	**HARDCORE MICROBIOLOGY**
Gram-Positive Bacteria			
Staphylococcus saprophyticus	• Gram-positive cocci in clusters • Coagulase − • Catalase + • Facultative anaerobe	Acute cystitis	Lactosamine residue adheres to the urothelium
Gram-Negative Bacteria			
Escherichia coli	• Gram-negative rod • Beta-hemolytic • Lactose fermenter • Indole + • Facultative anaerobe	Urinary tract infection, acute cystitis	Urinary tract infections can cause altered mental status in the elderly resembling delirium and dementia
Fungi			
Candida albicans	• Pseudohyphae and true hyphae • Oval-budding yeast	Vulvovaginal candidiasis	The most common cause of vulvovaginal candidiasis, Patients complain of a white, clumpy curd-like discharge, diagnosed by KOH preparation

TABLE 5-3	Musculoskeletal System		
BUGS	**BUG POINTS**	**MOST COMMON PRESENTATION**	**HARDCORE MICROBIOLOGY**
Gram-Positive Bacteria			
Staphylococcus aureus	• Gram-positive cocci (clusters) • Catalase + • Coagulase + • Beta-hemolytic	Osteomyelitis	Adheres to bone with adhesions; two toxins, exotoxin and toxic shock syndrome toxin (TSST-1); infects prosthetic joints

TABLE 5-4	Pulmonary System		
BUGS	**BUG POINTS**	**MOST COMMON PRESENTATION**	**HARDCORE MICROBIOLOGY**
Gram-Positive Bacteria			
Streptococcus pneumoniae	• Gram-positive, lancet-shaped diplococcus in chains • Catalase − • Ferments inulin • Optochin-sensitive • Alpha-hemolytic • Facultative anaerobe	Community-acquired, lobar pneumonia	Most common cause of community-acquired pneumonia
Gram-Negative Bacteria			
Chlamydia pneumoniae	• Gram-negative • Obligate	Lower respiratory tract infection, intracellular parasite	Interstitial infiltrates on CXR atypical pneumonia
Viruses			
Rhinovirus	• Single-stranded, RNA virus • *Picornaviridae*	Common cold	Spread with infected nasal secretions entering the nasopharynx through the nasal or ophthalmic mucosa

TABLE 5-5	Dermatological System		
BUGS	**BUG POINTS**	**MOST COMMON PRESENTATION**	**HARDCORE MICROBIOLOGY**
Gram-Positive Bacteria			
Staphylococcus aureus	• Gram-positive cocci (clusters) • Catalase + • Coagulase + • Beta-hemolytic	Furuncle, cellulitis	Commonly occurs patients who are obese, on corticosteroids, or who have deficient neutrophil function
Streptococcus pyogenes	• Gram-positive cocci in chains • Catalase – • Group A Lancefield • Facultative anaerobe	Cellulitis, erysipelas	Produces erythrogenic exotoxins, bactitracin sensitive, antibody to M proteins
Gram-Negative Bacteria			
Pseudomonas aeruginosa	• Gram-negative rod • Aerobe • Oxidase + • Nonlactose fermenter	"Hot tub" folliculitis	Occurs with exposure to whirlpools, swimming pools, and hot tubs contaminated with *Pseudomonas aeruginosa*
Viruses			
Human herpesvirus 7	• Linear double-stranded DNA virus	Pityriasis rosea	Replicates in CD4+ T lymphocytes, starts with "herald" patch lesion, develops in "Christmas tree" distribution
Varicella-zoster virus	• Double-stranded DNA virus • Herpesvirus alpha • Icosahedral nucleocapsid	Herpes-zoster (shingles)	Painful, unilateral vesicular eruption localized in a dermatomal distribution

CHAPTER 6

Infections of the Medical Student

Those of us in medical school are subjected to high levels of stress, long nights, and constant worry that make us more prone to certain types of infections than other people. Remember the following bugs if you encounter questions focused on this population.

Bugs discussed in this chapter:

- *Propionibacterium acnes*
- *Helicobacter pylori*
- *Epstein-Barr virus*

A. Gram-Positive Bacteria

Propionibacterium acnes

- Gram-positive rod
- Catalase +
- Aerobe

CLINICAL CORRELATES—ACNE VULGARIS

➤ *Propionibacterium acnes* is a normal component of the skin flora. In certain sebaceous glands, which are enlarged and *hyperresponsive to androgens*, this organism can proliferate, resulting in an *increased sebum production*.

➤ While proliferating in sebaceous glands, *P. acnes* releases chemotactic factors that attract neutrophils, and extrudes proinflammatory lipids and keratins into the surrounding dermis, causing irritation. When this irritation is combined with follicular hyperkeratinization, pimple formation occurs.

B. Gram-Negative Bacteria

Helicobacter pylori

- Gram-negative rod
- Urease +

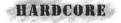

Chronic *H. pylori* infection is the most important risk factor for developing duodenal ulcer disease.

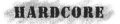

H. pylori should be treated with a triple regimen of either (1) bismuth, *metronidazole*, and *tetracycline*; or (2) proton pump inhibitor, *amoxicillin*, and *clarithromycin*.

CLINICAL CORRELATES—PEPTIC ULCER DISEASE, GASTRITIS

➤ The *H. pylori* organism is highly adapted for the gastric environment and exclusively *colonizes gastric-type epithelia*. Following colonization, *H. pylori* causes the disruption of the gastric mucosal layer; liberates enzymes and toxins, including the *H. pylori*-derived **cytotoxic protein** (encoded for by cytotoxin-associated gene A [CagA]); and adheres to the gastric epithelium, inciting a host immune response.

➤ The presence of *H. pylori* in the upper gastrointestinal tract is a significant risk factor for the development of **peptic ulcer disease**, and may contribute to the development of *gastric adenocarcinoma and primary B-cell lymphoma* of the stomach.

HARDCORE REVIEW TABLE—INFECTIONS OF THE MEDICAL STUDENTS (TABLE 6-1)

TABLE 6-1	Infections of the Medical Students		
BUGS	**BUG POINTS**	**MOST COMMON PRESENTATION**	**HARDCORE MICROBIOLOGY**
Gram-Positive Bacteria			
Propionibacterium acnes	• Gram-positive rod • Catalase + • Aerobe	Acne vulgaris	Part of normal skin flora
Gram-Negative Bacteria			
Helicobacter pylori	• Gram-negative rod • Urease +	PUD, gastritis	Colonizes gastric epithelium, urease breath test or gastric tissue biopsy used for diagnosis, seagull shaped
Viruses			
Epstein-Barr virus	• Double-stranded, linear DNA virus • Herpesvirus • Icosahedral nucleocapsid	Infectious mononucleosis ("kissing disease")	Spread by intimate contact, causes lymphocytosis with atypical lymphocytes, possibility of splenic rupture, diagnosis by heterophile antibody test

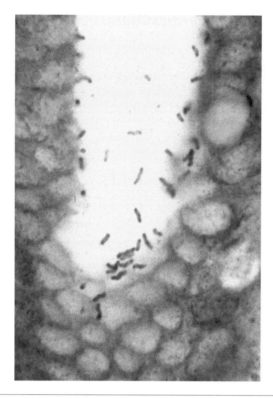

Figure 6-1 Infective gastritis. *Helicobacter pylori* appears on silver staining as small, curved rods on the surface of the gastric mucosa. *Reprinted with permission from Mitros FA: Atlas of Gastrointestinal Pathology. New York: Gower Medical Publishing, 1988.*

➤ A *urease breath test or gastric tissue biopsy* is used to identify the gastric presence of *H. pylori*.

➤ Under the microscope, *H. pylori* appears on silver staining as curved rods that resemble the *shape of a seagull* (Fig. 6-1).

C. Viruses

Epstein-Barr Virus

- Double-stranded, linear DNA virus
- Herpesvirus
- Icosahedral nucleocapsid

CLINICAL CORRELATES—INFECTIOUS MONONUCLEOSIS ("KISSING DISEASE")

➤ An Epstein-Barr viral infection results in the development of infectious mononucleosis, characterized by fatigue, high fever, tonsillar pharyngitis, lymphadenopathy, and splenomegaly. Typically, EBV is *spread by intimate contact* (via passage of saliva, or kissing) with a virus-shedding individual.

➤ Affected patients exhibit peripheral blood *lymphocytosis*, composed of *atypical lymphocytes* (CD8+ T-cells and CD16+ NK cells, but *not B-cells*) that may initially resemble a malignancy.

➤ A potentially serious complication of mononucleosis is *splenic rupture*, as these patients develop splenic expansion following lymphocytosis. Any young athelete should be told to avoid contact sports until the spleen returns to normal size.

➤ Diagnosis of EBV infection is made with a positive *heterophile antibody test* (*monospot*).

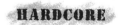

Mononucleosis can be precipitated by antibiotic use (*amoxicillin*).

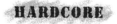

The EBV enters B-lymphocytes at the site of the C3 component of the complement system (C3d).

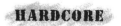

EBV may be associated with neurologic syndromes, including Guillain-Barré syndrome, facial nerve palsies, and meningoencephalitis.

CHAPTER 7

Infections of the Restaurant-Goer

When assessing the patient who presents with vomiting and diarrhea on Step 1, pay close attention to the type of diarrhea (watery or bloody), as well as the type of food consumed by the patient and the duration of time before symptoms started.

Bugs discussed in this chapter:

- *Bacillus cereus*
- *Staphylococcus aureus*
- *Campylobacter jejuni*
- *Escherichia coli*

- *Salmonella*
- *Shigella*
- *Vibrio parahaemolyticus*

A. Gram-Positive Bacteria

Bacillus cereus

- Gram-positive rod
- Aerobe
- Endospores

CLINICAL CORRELATES—GASTROENTERITIS

➤ *B. cereus* causes gastroenteritis after transfer to humans in *starchy foods such as rice*. This organism produces a preformed **heat-labile enterotoxin** (similar to that of cholergan, which inhibits sodium and chloride reabsorption) that induces a rapid (within 6 hours) onset of nausea and profuse vomiting. The disease is self-limited and the diagnosis is clinical.

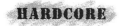

HARDCORE

B. cereus is classically associated with gastroenteritis after eating ***Chinese fried rice*** (Fig. 7-1).

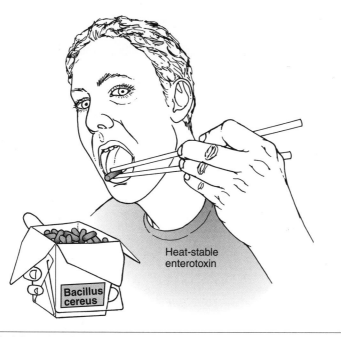

Heat-stable enterotoxin

Bacillus cereus

Figure 7-1 *B. cereus* is classically associated with gastroenteritis after eating ***Chinese fried rice***. Its preformed ***heat-stable*** *enterotoxin* causes a rapid onset of nausea and profuse vomiting.

Staphyloccus aureus

- Gram-positive cocci (clusters)
- Catalase +
- Coagulase +
- Beta-hemolytic

CLINICAL CORRELATES—STAPHYLOCOCCAL GASTROENTERITIS

➤ Food contaminated with *enterotoxin-producing* S. *aureus* results in acute vomiting and diarrhea within 4 to 6 hours of ingestion. Foods typically become contaminated by food handlers and improper refrigeration. Common foods include *egg salad, cream pastries, and coffee creamers.*

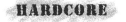

If acute gastroenteritis occurs soon after eating, *S. aureus* is the likely pathogen.

B. Gram-Negative Bacteria

Campylobacter jejuni

- Gram-negative rod
- Oxidase +

CLINICAL CORRELATES—CAMPYLOBACTER ENTERITIS

➤ *Campylobacter* infestation occurs in both the large and small intestine, causing acute mucosal inflammation with edema and crypt abscess formation resulting in *bloody, mucoid diarrhea.* After a prodrome of fever, rigors, dizziness, and possibly delirium, patients report frank blood in the stool by the third day of diarrhea. *Abdominal pain is more severe in Campylobacter enteritis than other bacterial diarrheas* and the organism may be excreted in the feces for several weeks after recovery.

➤ This organism inhabits the intestinal tracts of a wide range of animal hosts, notably *poultry,* and can be transmitted by consuming chicken, traveling to underdeveloped countries, drinking surface water, or drinking unpasterized milk.

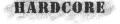

Campylobacter jejuni infection is a common infectious cause of *Guillain-Barré syndrome* (ascending paralysis).

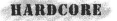

Pain from *Campylobacter* infection radiates to the right iliac fossa and can *mimic acute appendicitis*.

Escherichia coli

- Gram-negative rod
- Beta-hemolytic
- Lactose fermenter
- Indole +
- Facultative anaerobe

CLINICAL CORRELATES—DIARRHEA (WATERY AND BLOODY)

➤ Although *Escherichia coli* are normal inhabitants of the gastrointestinal tract, when E. *coli* strains acquire specific genetic material they can become pathogenic (Fig. 7-2). There are a number of types of E. *coli* identified, but the following are the most important:

- Enterohemorrhagic E. *coli* (EHEC)—Dominant *serotype O157:H7* produces a *Shiga-like exotoxin* that causes a copius, *bloody diarrhea* without mucosal invasion or inflammation. *Beef* is commonly the vehicle of transmission for E. *coli* O157:H7 infection.

- Enteroinvasive E. *coli* (EIEC)—EIEC invades epithelial cells causing *bloody diarrhea with WBCs* resembling shigellosis *in children* (same toxin as *Shigella*).

- Enterotoxigenic E. *coli* (ETEC)—ETEC is a significant cause of **traveler's diarrhea** spread by food or water contaminated with human waste. ETEC contains *heat-labile enterotoxins* that induce prolonged hypersecretion of chloride and water by intestinal mucosal cells, resulting in a severe, watery diarrhea.

- Enteropathogenic E. *coli* (EPEC)—EPEC causes *watery diarrhea in infants* by attaching to mucosal cells and destroying microvilli in the small intestine.

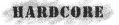

Shiga toxin can also cause systemic vascular damage resulting in hemolytic-uremic syndrome.

Salmonella

- Gram-negative rod
- Beta-hemolytic
- Non-lactose fermenter

CLINICAL CORRELATES—GASTROENTERITIS, TYPHOID FEVER

➤ *Salmonella* causes two broad categories of disease, typhoid and fever, and gastroenteritis.

1. *Typhoidal Salmonella* (S. *typhi* or S. *paratyphi*) cause a systemic illness not associated with diarrhea. Infection occurs via direct contact with an infected individual, or indirect contact

E. coli pathogenesis

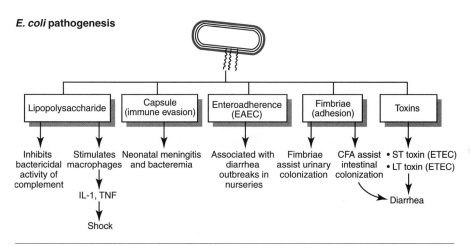

Figure 7-2 *E. coli* pathogenesis. *E. coli* infection causes sequelae in the host via several mechanisms including its extracellular capsule, LPS in its cell wall, its fimbriae that allow attachment to host cells, and multiple toxins depending on the strain of *E. coli* causing infection.

with **contaminated food or water.** Ingested organisms enter the lymphatic system and the bloodstream from the small intestine, resulting in high fever, rose spots on the skin, constipation, bradycardia, and potentially intestinal hemorrhage with perforation.

2. **Nontyphoidal Salmonella** (broad group) cause gastroenteritis characterized by nausea, vomiting, fever, and **bloody diarrhea with mucus** that develops within 72 hours of ingesting contaminated food or water. Transmission results from improperly handled food contaminated with fecal matter, most notably **eggs and poultry,** by fecal–oral contamination from other humans, or **pet animals, typically reptiles** (e.g., snakes, lizards, turtles, iguanas).

➤ *Salmonella* gains access to the submucosal region of the bowel by both directly penetrating epithelial cells and by attaching to specialized epithelial cells overlying Peyer's patches in the colon known as **M-cells.** These cells normally serve as a sampling and antigen-presenting cells in the mucosa lymphoid system.

Shigella

- Gram-negative rod
- Beta-hemolytic
- Non-lactose fermenter
- Indole +

CLINICAL CORRELATES—BACTERIAL DIARRHEA

➤ *Shigella* is a pathogen that invades colonic enterocytes, resulting in **bloody, mucoid diarrhea.** Patients with *Shigella* gastroenteritis present with high fever, abdominal cramps, and eventually mucus and blood in their diarrhea. Transmission of this bacterium occurs by both direct person-to-person spread and from contaminated food and water.

Vibrio parahaemolyticus

- Gram-negative rod
- Oxidase +
- Ferments sugars except lactose

CLINICAL CORRELATES—DIARRHEA

➤ *V. parahaemolyticus* is a cause of **seafood-associated** (raw fish and shellfish) diarrhea (Fig. 7-3). This organism grows well on blood agar and other nonselective media.

C. Viruses

Hepatitis A

- Positive, single-stranded RNA virus
- *Picornaviridae*
- Icosahedral capsid

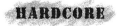

After acute *Salmonella* infection, 1% to 4% of individuals will become chronic, asymptomatic carriers of *S. typhi*. Under unsanitary conditions, these asymptomatic carriers can pass the organism to many other people. This is best exemplified by "typhoid Mary," a cook in the early 1900s in New York City who was an asymptomatic *S. typhi* carrier and eventually infected approximately 50 people (three fatally) with typhoid fever.

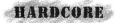

Salmonella infection may lead to hypertrophy of Peyer's patches via recruitment of mononuclear cells and lymphocytes.

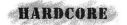

Salmonella differs from *Shigella* in that it is motile, but not as virulent.

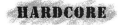

Nausea and vomiting are absent in most patients with *Shigella* infection.

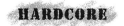

Shigella is very virulent; as few as 10 *Shigella* organisms can cause infection.

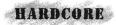

There are four types of *Shigella*: *boydii*, *dysenteriae*, *flexneri*, and *sonnei*. *S. sonnei* accounts for more than two thirds of shigellosis cases in the United States; almost all the rest are from *S. flexneri*. *S. dysenteriae* is rare in the United States but important in developing countries.

HARDCORE

Shigella has **no animal reservoir!** It is transmitted by food and human contact.

HARDCORE

V. parahaemolyticus is **comma-shaped with a single flagellum.**

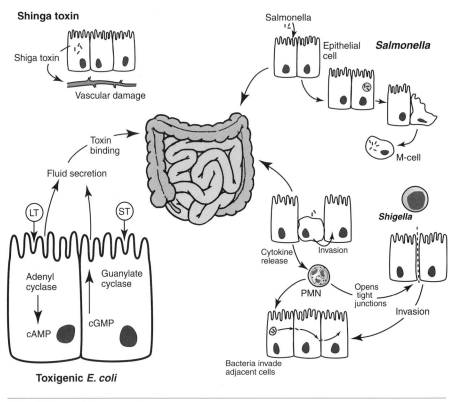

Figure 7-3 Overview of diarrhea caused by bacteria.

CLINICAL CORRELATES—HEPATITIS A INFECTION

➤ Hepatitis A infection results in an acute illness acquired by consuming contaminated food, most commonly from uncooked *shellfish* (raw oysters). The virus spreads via the *fecal–oral route* and results in vomiting, fever, and right upper quadrant pain, as well as potential symptoms of hepatitis including dark urine, acholic stool, jaundice, and pruritus.

➤ There is no antigenic cross-reactivity to HAV with HBV or HCV.

➤ Remember that hepatitis A infection is an acute, self-limited illness.

HARDCORE REVIEW TABLES—INFECTIONS OF THE RESTAURANT-GOER (TABLE 7-1 TO TABLE 7-6)

TABLE 7-1	Bloody Diarrhea Hardcore Points
ORGANISMS THAT CAUSE BLOODY DIARRHEA	
Campylobacter	Transmitted in poultry; abdominal pain is more severe than in other bacterial diarrheas
Shigella	Nausea and vomiting are absent; no animal reservoir so acquired by direct person-to-person spread
Salmonella typhi	Transmitted in eggs and poultry or via pet reptiles
Enteroinvasive *E. coli*	Invades epithelial cells, causing bloody diarrhea with WBC that resembles shigellosis in children
Enterohemorrhagic *E. coli*	Serotype O157:H7 produces a Shiga-like exotoxin but no mucosal invasion or inflammation; transmitted in beef

TABLE 7-2	Common Pathogen (Gastroenteritis) by Food Item
Poultry products	*Campylobacter jejuni*
Custard and potato salad	*Staphylococcus aureus*
Carriers	*Salmonella typhi*
Milk and cream	*Listeria* or *Mycobacterium bovis*

(Continued)

TABLE 7-2 | Common Pathogen (Gastroenteritis) by Food Item (cont.)

Poorly canned green vegetables	*Clostridium botulinum*
Poorly washed salad greens	*E. coli, Entamoeba histolytica, Salmonella, Shigella*
Rare red meat dishes	*E. coli* or *Trichinella spiralis*
Rice dishes	*Bacillus cereus*
Smoked fish	*Clostridium botulinum*
Raw eggs	*Salmonella*
Raw seafood	*Vibrio, Norovirus,* hepatitis A
Uncooked shellfish (raw oysters)	Hepatitis A
Undercooked meat	*Salmonella, Cambylobacter,* ETEC
Soft cheeses	*Listeria monocytogenes*

TABLE 7-3 | Presenting Symptoms of Common Food-Borne Microbes

PRESENTING SYMPTOM	COMMON PATHOGENS	POSSIBLE FOOD SOURCE	TIME PERIOD TO SYMPTOMS
Watery diarrhea	ETEC Enteric viruses	Fecally contaminated food/water Fecally contaminated food/water	1–3 days 1–3 days
Inflammatory diarrhea	*Camplyobacter Salmonella* *Shigella* toxin-producing *E. coli Shigella* *V. parahaemolyticus*	Poultry, unpasteurized milk Eggs, poultry, meat, unpasteurized milk Ground beef, raw vegetables Fecally contaminated food/water Raw shellfish	2–5 days 1–3 days 1–7 days 1–3 days Within 2 days
Vomiting	*S. aureus* *B. cereus* Norwalk-like viruses	Prepared food Rice, meat Shellfish, prepared food	Within 6 hours Within 6 hours 1–2 days

TABLE 7-4 | Gram-Positive Bacteria

BUGS	BUG POINTS	MOST COMMON PRESENTATION	HARDCORE MICROBIOLOGY
Bacillus cereus	• Gram-positive rod • Aerobe • Endospores	Gastroenteritis	Associated with eating Chinese fried rice, nausea within 6 hours, produces a preformed heat-stable enterotoxin
Staphylococcus aureus	• Gram-positive cocci (clusters) • Catalase + • Coagulase + • Beta-hemolytic	Staphylococcal gastroenteritis ○ Acute vomiting ○ Diarrhea	Symptoms within 4–6 hours of ingestion; typically contaminated food include egg salad, cream pastries, and coffee creamers

TABLE 7-5 | Gram-Negative Bacteria

BUGS	BUG POINTS	MOST COMMON PRESENTATION	HARDCORE MICROBIOLOGY
Campylobacter jejuni	• Gram-negative rod • Oxidase +	*Campylobacter* enteritis ○ Mucoid, bloody diarrhea	Transmitted by consuming chicken, drinking surface water in underdeveloped countries, drinking raw milk
Escherichia coli	• Gram-negative rod • Beta-hemolytic • Lactose fermenter • Indole + • Facultative anaerobe	Diarrhea ○ Watery and bloody	• *Enterohemorrhagic* E. coli *(EHEC)*—dominant serotype O157:H7 produces a Shiga-like exotoxin causing a copius, bloody diarrhea without mucosal invasion or inflammation. Beef is commonly the vehicle of transmission • *Enteroinvasive* E. coli *(EIEC)*—causes bloody diarrhea with WBC, same toxin as *Shigella* • *Enterotoxigenic* E. coli *(ETEC)*—significant cause of traveler's diarrhea spread by food or water contaminated with human waste. Contains heat-labile and heat-stable enterotoxins that cause prolonged hypersecretion of chloride and waterby intestinal mucosal cells • *Enteropathogenic* E. coli *(EPEC)*—causes watery diarrhea in infants

(Continued)

TABLE 7-5 Gram-Negative Bacteria (cont.)

Bugs	Bug Points	Most Common Presentation	Hardcore Microbiology
Salmonella	• Gram-negative rod • Beta-hemolytic • Non-lactose fermenter	Gastroenteritis ○ Vomiting ○ Fever ○ Bloody, mucoid diarrhea	Symptoms develop within 72 hours, transmission via eggs and poultry and reptile pets, may lead to hypertrophy of Peyer's patches
Shigella dysenteriae	• Gram-negative rod • Beta-hemolytic • Non-lactose fermenter • Indole +	Bacterial diarrhea ○ Bloody, mucoid diarrhea with pus	Spread via fecal–oral route
Vibrio parahaemolyticus	• Gram-negative rod • Oxidase + • Ferments sugars except lactose	Diarrhea	Seafood associated (raw fish and shellfish), grows on blood agar

TABLE 7-6 Viruses

Bugs	Bug Points	Most Common Presentation	Hardcore Microbiology
Hepatitis A	• Positive, single-stranded RNA virus • *Picornaviridae* • Icosahedral capsid	Acute hepatitis A infection	• Acquired fecal–oral • Typically from uncooked shellfish (raw oysters) • Can develop symptoms of hepatitis including dark urine, acholic stool, jaundice, and pruritus

CHAPTER 8

Infections of Hospitalized Patients

As a physician, you will of course be treating a lot of infections in hospitalized patients, which is why Step 1 will test you on the bugs that cause them. Hospitalized patients often are infected by organisms that do not typically afflict the healthy community-dweller. Focus on the various signs of infection and sepsis in the hospitalized patient in addition to the classic organisms that cause infection in each organ system.

Bugs discussed in this chapter:

- *Staphylococcus aureus*
- *Staphylococcus epidermidis*
- *Streptococcus viridans*
- *Enterococcus*
- *Escherichia coli*
- *Candida*
- *Pseudomonas aeruginosa*
- *Legionella pneumophila*

- *Clostridium difficile*
- *Bacteroides fragilis*
- *Proteus mirabilis*
- *Klebsiella pneumoniae*
- *Serratia marcescens*
- *Staphylococcus pyogenes*
- *Clostridium perfringens*

I. CARDIOVASCULAR SYSTEM

Endocarditis is the most important infection to consider in the cardiovascular system in a hospitalized patient, and is most commonly caused by gram-positive bacteria. This disease is characterized by an infection of the endocardium, or, more commonly, the heart valve leaflets or walls. Endocarditis may be acute or subacute determined by the following:

- *Acute bacterial endocarditis (ABE)*—Infection of previously healthy valves that typically causes metastatic foci and is generally fatal if not treated within 6 weeks.
  - Common organism: *Staphylococcus aureus*.
- *Subacute bacterial endocarditis (SBE)*—A seeding of previously damaged valves that does not produce metastatic foci.
  - Common organism: *Streptococcus viridans* and *Staphylococcus epidermidis* (prosthetic valves).

Staphylococcus aureus

- Gram-positive cocci (clusters)
- Catalase +
- Coagulase +
- Beta-hemolytic

CLINICAL CORRELATES—ACUTE BACTERIAL ENDOCARDITIS

➤ Most commonly affects previously normal heart valves. This infection can lead to **metastatic foci** of infectious *S. aureus* to the lungs (right-sided ABE), brain (left-sided ABE), and other end organs (if the left heart is infected).

➤ Look for the association of ABE with **intravenous drug abuse (IVDA)** on boards.

Staphylococcus epidermidis

- Gram-positive cocci (clusters)
- Catalase +
- Coagulase –
- Facultative anaerobe

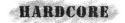

HARDCORE

S. aureus is the **main coagulase (+)** **Staphylococcus species**.

CLINICAL CORRELATES—SUBACUTE ENDOCARDITIS OF PROSTHETIC HEART VALVES

➤ This bug's polysaccharide capsule allows it to adhere to prosthetic devices, including *prosthetic heart valves*. *S. epidermidis* lives normally on our skin and can gain access into the bloodstream via IV catheters and other invasive devices.

Streptococcus viridans

- Gram-positive cocci (chains)
- Catalase –
- Coagulase –
- Facultative anaerobe

CLINICAL CORRELATES—SUBACUTE BACTERIAL ENDOCARDITIS (SBE)

➤ *S. viridans* causes a low-grade infection that is difficult to diagnose because of its nonspecific symptoms (*increased fatigue and a new heart murmur*). Typically, this bug *seeds previously damaged heart valves* from rheumatic heart disease or congenital heart defects, including mitral valve prolapse.

➤ *S. viridans* is part of the normal oral flora. It is *alpha-hemolytic but optochin resistant*, differentiating it from *Streptococcus pneumoniae*, which is alpha-hemolytic but optochin-sensitive

II. HEMATOLOGICAL SYSTEM

The term **bacteremia** refers to the presence of viable bacteria in the normally sterile bloodstream. Bacteremia within the hospital setting may be caused by either direct infection (primary) or by secondary infections. Secondary infections are related to infections at other sites, such as the urinary tract, lung, postoperative wounds, and skin. Bacterial hematologic infections are an important cause of morbidity and mortality within the hospital population because they may result in the development of *sepsis* and *septic shock*:

- **Sepsis** refers to the systemic, *widespread inflammatory response* to an infection characterized by fever, elevated heart rate, increased respiratory rate, and an increased white blood cell count.
- **Septic shock** is sepsis *with hypotension* despite having an adequate fluid status. Sepsis may result in shock if the inflammatory reaction is widespread enough to result in a marked reduction in systemic vascular resistance and compensatory increase in cardiac output.

A. Gram-Positive Bacteria

Staphylococcus aureus

- Gram-positive cocci (clusters)
- Catalase +
- Coagulase +
- Beta-hemolytic

CLINICAL CORRELATES—SEPSIS

➤ *Staphylococcus aureus* is the leading cause of both *community-acquired* and *hospital-acquired bacteremia*.

➤ Approximately 20% to 30% of hospitalized patients with Staph-induced bacteremia will die from the infection.

Enterococci (*E. faecalis* and *E. faecium*)

- Gram-positive cocci (chains)
- Lancefield group D
- Facultative anaerobe

CLINICAL CORRELATES—SEPSIS

➤ Enterococci are becoming a serious infectious organism primarily because they possess a diverse resistance profile to many commonly used antibiotics (including *penicillins, cephalosporins, and vancomycin*).

➤ Resistant strains of **vancomycin-resistant enterococci (VRE)** include phenotypes VanA–VanG, in which each phenotype carries variable levels of resistance.

➤ Enterococci are part of the normal intestinal and oral flora in humans and animals.

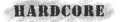

S. epidermidis infection is associated with foreign objects and invasive devices, so when you hear prosthetic valve and endocarditis in the same sentence, the organism is usually *S. epidermidis*.

HARDCORE

S. epidermidis **does not make coagulase**, while *S. aureus* does.

HARDCORE

S. viridans typically causes **subacute** bacterial endocarditis, while *S. aureus* typically causes **acute** bacterial endocarditis.

Remember that **VIR**idans is **VIR**tuous and will not kill you (it is subacute)!

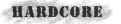

Gram-negative sepsis is much more serious and rapidly developing than grampositive sepsis; intervention in these patients must be immediate.

B. Gram-Negative Bacteria

Escherichia coli

- Gram-negative rod
- Beta-hemolytic
- Lactose fermenter
- Indole +
- Facultative anaerobe

CLINICAL CORRELATES—SEPSIS

➤ When normal host defenses are diminished, such as in the hospitalized patient, E. coli can reach the bloodstream, resulting in sepsis. Typically, this follows an untreated urinary tract infection.

C. Fungi

Candida species

- Pseudohyphae and true hyphae
- Oval-budding yeast

CLINICAL CORRELATES—SEPSIS, CANDIDEMIA

➤ **Candidemia** indicates the presence of a *Candida* species in the bloodstream. Typically, these infections are seen in hospitalized and immunosuppressed patients (**ICU and HIV patients**).

➤ Diagnosis of candidemia requires **KOH stain** and a blood culture looking for the presence of **pseudohyphae or true hyphae**.

III. PULMONARY SYSTEM

A. Gram-Positive Bacteria

Staphylococcus aureus

- Gram-positive cocci (clusters)
- Catalase +
- Coagulase +
- Beta-hemolytic

CLINICAL CORRELATES—PNEUMONIA, LUNG CAVITATIONS, EFFUSIONS, EMPYEMAS (PUS IN THE PLEURAL SPACE), AND ABSCESSES

➤ S. *aureus* can directly invade the lungs via its virulence factor, **protein A**. Protein A is located on its cell membrane and **binds to the Fc portion of host IgG, inhibiting complement fixation**. This disarms a portion of the immune system defense and can result in a nasty pneumonia characterized by **lobar consolidation**.

➤ Some S. *aureus* organisms have become resistant to the antibiotic **methicillin** due to the overuse of broad-spectrum antibiotics in the hospital. This strain of S. *aureus* is called **methicillin-resistant Staphylococcus aureus (MRSA)**. When these resistant organisms cause pneumonia (or any infection), they are extremely difficult to treat because they are only susceptible to antibiotic treatment with a select few agents.

B. Gram-Negative Bacteria

Pseudomonas aeruginosa

- Gram-negative rod
- Aerobe
- Oxidase +
- Non-lactose fermenter

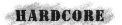

HARDCORE

E. coli is the most **common cause of gram-negative sepsis**. *Klebsiella* and *Pseudomonas* are other causes.

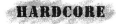

HARDCORE

The lactose fermenters include *E. coli, Citrobacter, Enterobacter, Klebsiella,* and *Serratia*.

HARDCORE

Newborns are highly susceptible to *E. coli* sepsis because they **lack IgM antibodies**.

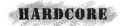

HARDCORE

The presence of fungi in any blood culture is never a contaminant and should always be taken as a serious infection.

CLINICAL CORRELATES—PNEUMONIA

➢ The *Pseudomonas* organism is only weakly invasive, and therefore usually infects only the most sick people in the hospital. Typically, this includes those in the ICU, burn victims, and patients who are immunocompromised (cystic fibrosis patients).

➢ The major virulence factor of *Pseudomonas* is *exotoxin A*, which is an ADP-ribose transferase that inhibits protein synthesis by inhibiting EF-2 (*same as the diphtheria toxin*). In addition, the *Pseudomonas* organism possesses an *exoenzyme S*, which also inhibits protein synthesis, an *endotoxin* that triggers inflammation, and several *proteolytic enzymes*.

➢ When cultured, *Pseudomonas* forms a *blue-green—colored colony* and has a *fruity odor*.

Legionella pneumophila

- Gram-negative rod
- Catalase +
- Beta-lactase +
- Facultative intracellular parasite
- Aerobic

CLINICAL CORRELATES—LEGIONNAIRE'S DISEASE

➢ *Legionella* lives in water sources (like *air conditioning systems*) and can be aerosolized and inhaled, leading to *Legionnaire's disease*. Legionnaire's causes high fever and severe pneumonia in hospitalized patients.

➢ Suspect *Legionella* in a patient *over 50 years old when a sputum Gram stain only reveals a few organisms* (because *Legionella* is *intracellular*). Serology confirms the diagnosis (ELISA or a urine antigen test).

➢ *Legionella inhibits phagosome–lysosome fusion*, and may be phagocytosed by macrophages without being killed! It can live inside macrophages and replicate. Use a *silver stain* to see the small organisms, or grow *Legionella* on *charcoal yeast agar* (Fig. 8-1).

HARDCORE

Legionnaire's disease is named for the outbreak of pneumonia caused by *Legionella* in 1976 at an American Legion convention in Philadelphia.

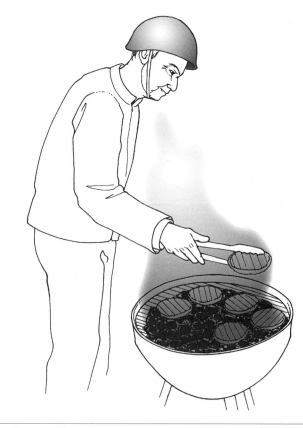

Figure 8–1 Pneumonia-causing *Legionella* is diagnosed with a **silver** stain or grown on a **charcoal** yeast agar. *Think of an old soldier, a knight of the American legion wearing a silver helmet (silver stain) while tending the charcoal (charcoal yeast agar) on his bareque.*

IV. GASTROINTESTINAL SYSTEM

The main GI complication in the hospitalized patient is *diarrhea*. Watch out primarily for *Clostridium difficile*, which causes severe diarrhea, abdominal cramps, and fever following a course of routine antibiotics, specifically *clindamycin*, and other broad-spectrum antibiotics. Antibiotics wipe out the normal flora in the colon, allowing *C. difficile* to proliferate and cause infection.

A. Gram-Positive Bacteria

Clostridium difficile

- Gram-positive rod
- Anaerobe
- Endospores

CLINICAL CORRELATES—PSEUDOMEMBRANOUS ENTEROCOLITIS

➤ *C. difficile* causes **pseudomembranous enterocolitis**, named for a white exudative pseudomembrane the organism causes on the surface of the large intestine. This pseudomembrane can be visualized by colonoscopy, demonstrating *mucosal necrosis beneath the pseudomembrane*.

➤ *C. difficile* is a belligerent bug because of its virulence factors:

○ *Exotoxin A* causes diarrhea, while *exotoxin B* is cytotoxic to mucosal cells. For diagnosis, test for the presence of *C. difficile* toxin on a stool sample.

○ **Endospores** are a form of metabolically dormant, heat-resistant bacteria. They can become activated when exposed to a favorable environment, and they can only be killed by auto-clave. These endospores therefore are able to survive in the hospital environment and when ingested (fecal–oral), they cause diarrhea.

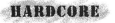

C. difficile diarrhea typically follows a course of the antibiotic *clindamycin*.

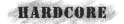

Endospores are only produced by two genera of bacteria, *Bacillus* and *Clostridium*.

B. Gram-Negative Bacteria

Bacteroides fragilis

- Gram-negative enteric rod
- Obligate anaerobic

CLINICAL CORRELATES—ABSCESS FORMATION

➤ *B. fragilis* is a normal component of the GI tract. However, if this bug gains access to the peritoneal cavity through trauma, infection, or a surgical complication, it can result in an abscess formation that leads to bacteremia and sepsis.

➤ This organism is *obligate anaerobic* and contains a *polysaccharide capsule*, but *no endotoxin*.

V. GENITOURINARY SYSTEM

Urinary tract infections (UTIs) in hospitalized patients are commonly caused by the insertion of instrumentation into the vagina or urethra, which introduces bacteria into the normally sterile urinary tract. In the hospitalized patient, this means the insertion of *in-dwelling urinary catheters* (Foley catheter). Gram-negative organisms are the most common bugs isolated from the urine of a catheterized patient, including *E. coli*, *Proteus*, *Klebsiella*, *Serratia*, and *Pseudomonas*.

Escherichia coli

- Gram-negative rod
- Beta-hemolytic
- Lactose fermenter
- Indole +
- Facultative anaerobe

CLINICAL CORRELATES—UTI

➤ *E. coli is the most common cause of UTI*. *E coli's* **pili** enable the bug to adhere to— and ascend up— the urinary tract.

➤ Typical symptoms of *E. coli* UTI include a burning sensation while urinating, the need to urinate more frequently, and an urgency to urinate.

Abscesses typically cannot be treated with antibiotics and must be drained surgically or percutaneously.

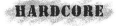

E. coli is an especially common cause of UTIs in females due to the close proximity of the anus to the vagina (*E. coli* normally colonizes the colon).

Proteus mirabilis

- Gram-negative rod
- Lactose fermenter

CLINICAL CORRELATES—UREASE-POSITIVE UTI

➤ This organism is characterized by a **tumbling motility** that has been described as "swarms" on **agar** when cultured. In addition, *Proteus* is distinguished by its production of **urease**, which is the same enzyme that causes a positive reaction on the *H. pylori* urease breath test for peptic ulcer disease.

➤ Urinalysis in patients with a suspected *Proteus* UTI will reveal an **alkaline pH** due to *Proteus'* ability to **split urea** into NH_3 and CO_2.

➤ *Proteus* infection may be associated with **struvite stones** (staghorn calculi) in patients with renal calculi.

Klebsiella pneumoniae

- Gram-negative rod
- Lactose fermenter
- Enteric bacteria

CLINICAL CORRELATES—UTI

➤ *Klebsiella* UTI will present much like infections caused by other organisms, which means it requires a urine culture to confirm its presence.

➤ This bug is encapsulated with an O-antigen capsule and forms **mucoid colonies on agar**.

Serratia marcescens

- Gram-negative rod
- Lactose fermenter

CLINICAL CORRELATES—UTI

➤ *S. marcescens* is a rare form of UTI that is classically differentiated from other bugs because it produces a **red pigment**.

- Remember, *Serratia* is **red**, similar to your **blood** when you cut yourself with a **serrated** knife.

Pseudomonas aeruginosa

- Gram-negative rod
- Aerobe
- Oxidase +
- Non-lactose fermenter

CLINICAL CORRELATES—UTI

➤ *Pseudomonas* likes water, has a **blue-green pigment**, and has a fruity smell (Fig. 8-2).

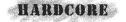

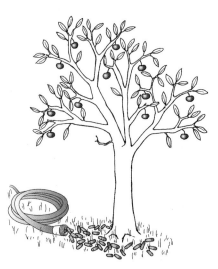

Figure 8–2 *Pseudomonas AlRuginosa* is bluish, like AIR and water, and smells like fruit (from a fruit tree), which needs AIR and water to grow.

VI. SKIN

When you think about the organisms that cause skin infections, think about the normal flora that live on skin: *Staph and Strep*. In hospitalized patients, *Clostridium perfringens* also poses a unique threat. Hospital-acquired wound infections are mostly seen after surgery, so in a scenario of *immediate postoperative fever*, think of two bugs first: *C. perfringens* and Group A *Streptococcus* (aka *S. pyogenes*).

Clostridium perfringens

- Gram-positive rod
- Anaerobe
- Endospores

CLINICAL CORRELATES—MYONECROSIS AND EARLY POSTOPERATIVE WOUND INFECTION

➤ *C. perfringens* produces *alpha toxin*, which is a hemolytic lecithinase. This virulence factor allows *Clostridium* to eat through tissues, resulting in myonecrosis, which presents as a *"dish water discharge"* within 24 hours after surgery. This is typically accompanied by exquisite pain and the formation of gas under the skin creating crepitus when palpated (*gas gangrene*).

➤ This infection requires multiple antibiotics and *aggressive surgical debridement* immediately after its diagnosis.

Staphylococcus aureus

- Gram-positive cocci (clusters)
- C+
- Coagulase +
- Beta-hemolytic

CLINICAL CORRELATES—CELLULITIS, ERYSIPELAS, IMPETIGO, AND SCALDED SKIN SYNDROME

➤ In contrast to *S. pyogenes*, *S. aureus* typically causes more subacute wound infections. *S. aureus* (as well as streptococcal) skin infections include *cellulitis, erysipelas, and impetigo*, but may also be responsible for the staphylococcal *scalded skin syndrome*, which is characterized by an extensive sloughing of skin.

➤ The virulence factors of *S. aureus* include *protein A* and the *TSST-1 toxin*, which acts as a *superantigen*. This toxin binds to class II MHC on host T-cells, but does not dissociate, resulting in continuous activation of T-cells and the inflammation cascade and the development of *toxic shock syndrome*.

- **Methicillin-resistant** *Staphylococcus aureus* **(MRSA)** causes the same skin infections as its more benign cousin *S. aureus*, but unfortunately is much more difficult to treat.
  - ○ MRSA is resistant to penicillin-family antibiotics because this bug possesses a special gene, *mecA*. The mecA gene encodes a protein called the *penicillin-binding protein 2a* (PBP2a). Normal (methicillin-sensitive) *S. aureus* contains PBPs in its cytoplasmic membrane, which are targets for beta-lactam antibiotics, and the inactivation of these PBPs leads to bacterial death. PBP2a does not bind beta-lactam antibiotics and therefore results in an *S. aureus* resistant to antibiotics that function by this mechanism.

Streptococcus pyogenes

- Gram-positive cocci in chains
- Catalase –
- Group A Lancefield
- Facultative anaerobe

CLINICAL CORRELATES—NECROTIZING FASCIITIS

➤ This is the most common cause of the famous *"flesh-eating bacteria,"* or in medical talk, **necrotizing fasciitis**, a favorite of the USMLE. Clinically, it is more commonly seen in diabetic patients and is associated with extreme pain and a reddish purple area that often forms *bullae or large blisters*; however, this infection may initially present only as an area of cutaneous erythema. Systemic signs include fever and hypotension.

- ▪ Think of fiery Strep **PYRO**genes, like a **PYRO**manic setting forest fires. It causes necrotizing fasciitis, which spreads dangerously through the skin *like flames*.

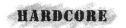

Remember the important anaerobes!

Cool **B**acteria are **A**naerobes—**C**lostridium, **B**acteroides, **A**ctinomyces (*C, B, A*)

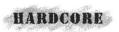

S. aureus is the most common organism found in wound infections.

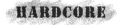

A description of a patient with sloughing skin should prompt you to think of two possibilities:

- If the question is asking for an organism responsible for such a presentation, the answer is *S. aureus* causing scalded skin syndrome (caused by the exfoliatin toxin).
- The second possibility is a drug reaction called *Stevens-Johnson Syndrome/ toxic epidermal necrolysis*, which can present very similarly—aminopenicillins (amoxicillin, ampicillin) are a common offender.

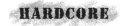

Scalded skin syndrome is most common in children, and Stevens-Johnson Syndrome is a disease of adults.

HARDCORE REVIEW TABLES—INFECTIONS OF HOSPITALIZED PATIENTS (TABLE 8-1 TO TABLE 8-6)

TABLE 8-1	Cardiovascular System		
BUGS	BUG POINTS	MOST COMMON PRESENTATION	HARDCORE MICROBIOLOGY
Gram-Positive Bacteria			
Staphylococcus aureus	• Gram-positive cocci (clusters) • Catalase + • Coagulase + • Beta-hemolytic	Acute bacterial endocarditis	Mostly seen in intravenous drug abuse (IVDA)
Staphylococcus epidermidis	• Gram-positive cocci (clusters) • Catalase + • Coagulase – • Facultative anaerobe	Subacute bacterial endocarditis	Patents with prosthetic heart valves
Streptococcus viridans	• Gram-positive cocci (chains) • Catalase – • Coagulase – • Facultative anaerobe	Subacute bacterial endocarditis	No Lancefield antigen

TABLE 8-2	Hematological System		
BUGS	BUG POINTS	MOST COMMON PRESENTATION	HARDCORE MICROBIOLOGY
Gram-Positive Bacteria			
Staphylococcus aureus	• Gram-positive cocci (clusters) • Catalase + • Coagulase + • Beta-hemolytic	Bacteremia, sepsis, and septic shock	Leading cause of community- and hospital-acquired bacteremia
Enterococci	• Gram-positive cocci (chains) • Lancefield group D • Facultative anaerobe	Bacteremia, sepsis, and septic shock	Strains of vancomycin-resistant enterococci (VRE) becoming more common
Gram-Negative Bacteria			
Escherichia coli	• Gram-negative rod • Beta-hemolytic • Lactose fermenter • Indole + • Facultative anaerobe	Bacteremia, sepsis, and septic shock	Rapidly progresses to septic shock
Fungals			
Candida species	• Pseudohyphae and true hyphae • Oval-budding yeast	Bacteremia, sepsis, and septic shock	Often in an immunocompromised host

TABLE 8-3	Pulmonary System		
BUGS	BUG POINTS	MOST COMMON PRESENTATION	HARDCORE MICROBIOLOGY
Gram-Positive Bacteria			
Staphylococcus aureus	• Gram-positive cocci (clusters) • Catalase + • Coagulase + • Beta-hemolytic	Lobar consolidation pneumonia abscesses, lung cavitations, effusions, empyemas, and abscesses	Contains the virulence factor protein A, which inhibits host opsonization and phagocytosis by IgG
Gram-Negative Bacteria			
Pseudomonas aeruginosa	• Gram-negative rod • Aerobe • Oxidase + • Non-lactose fermenter	Pneumonia	Often in an immunocompromised host; blue-green, fruity odor
Legionella pneumophila	• Gram-negative rod • Catalase + • Beta-lactase + • Facultative intracellular parasite	Legionnaire's disease: pneumonia and high fever	Source is typically associated with an air-conditioning unit or anything that aerosolyzes water

TABLE 8-4	Gastrointestinal System		
BUGS	**BUG POINTS**	**MOST COMMON PRESENTATION**	**HARDCORE MICROBIOLOGY**
Gram-Positive Bacteria			
Clostridium difficile	• Gram-positive rod • Anaerobe • Endospores	Pseudomembranous enterocolitis	Typically follows course of antibiotics (clindamycin)
Gram-Negative Bacteria			
Bacteroides fragilis	• Gram-negative enteric rod • Anaerobic	Abdominal abcess	Normal component of GI tract No endotoxin, but does have a polysaccharide capsule

TABLE 8-5	Genitourinary System		
BUGS	**BUG POINTS**	**MOST COMMON PRESENTATION**	**HARDCORE MICROBIOLOGY**
Gram-Negative Bacteria			
Escherichia coli	• Gram-negative rod • Beta-hemolytic • Lactose fermenter • Indole + • Facultative anaerobe	Most common cause of urinary tract infections	Pili enable *E. coli* to adhere to ascend the urinary tract
Proteus mirabilis	• Gram-negative rod • Lactose fermenter	Urinary tract infection	Associated with struvite stones (staghorn calculi); use agar plate; alkaline pH
Klebsiella pneumoniae	• Gram-negative rod • Lactose fermenter • Enteric bacteria	Urinary tract infection	Forms mucoid colonies on agar
Serratia marcescens	• Gram-negative rod • Lactose fermenter	Urinary tract infection	Red pigment
Pseudomonas aeruginosa	• Gram-negative rod • Aerobe • Oxidase + • Non-lactose fermenter	Urinary tract infection	Blue-green pigment

TABLE 8-6	Skin		
BUGS	**BUG POINTS**	**MOST COMMON PATHOLOGIC PRESENTATION**	**HARDCORE MICROBIOLOGY**
Gram-Positive Bacteria			
Clostridium perfringens	• Gram-positive rod • Anaerobe • Endospores	Myonecrosis	Dish water discharge
Group A *Streptococcus* (*S. pyogenes*)	• Gram-positive cocci in chains • Catalase – • Group A Lancefield • Facultative anaerobe	Necrotizing fasciitis	Bullae or large blisters
Staphylococcus aureus	• Gram-positive cocci (clusters) • Catalase + • Coagulase + • Beta-hemolytic	Cellulitis, erysipelas, impetigo, scaled skin syndrome, toxic shock syndrome	TSST-1 toxin and virulence factor protein A

CHAPTER 9

Infections of Immunocompromised Patients

Immunocompromised patients represent a unique population in which certain infectious organisms are routinely encountered, especially on USMLE exams. Be on the lookout for patients undergoing treatments for malignancy (neutropenic), patients following solid organ and bone marrow transplantation, patients with human immunodeficiency virus/acquired immunodeficiency syndrome (HIV/AIDS), and patients with dysfunctional splenic function for the following bugs (Fig. 9-1):

Bugs discussed in this chapter:

- HIV
- *Listeria*
- *Mycobacterium tuberculosis*
- *Mycobacterium avium*
- *Mycobacterium intracellulare*
- *Cytomegalovirus*
- Human herpesvirus 8
- JC virus
- *Pneumocystis carinii*
- *Aspergillus*

- *Cryptococcus neoformans*
- *Toxoplasma gondii*
- *Streptococcus pneumoniae*
- *Haemophilus influenzae*
- *Neisseria meningitidis*
- *Salmonella*
- *Parvovirus* B 19
- *Pseudomonas aeruginosa*
- *Cryptosporidium*

I. HUMAN IMMUNODEFICIENCY VIRUS

- Retrovirus
- Lentivirus

CLINICAL CORRELATES—HIV

➤ **Human immunodeficiency virus (HIV)** is a retrovirus that attacks lymphocytes and other cells expressing the **CD4 surface protein**. HIV gradually depletes the body of CD4 lymphocytes (Th1), creating an ideal environment for opportunistic pathogens. As the disease progresses and the CD4 count drops, the infected individual may eventually succumb to any of the opportunistic infectious organisms described in this chapter (Fig. 9-2).

➤ HIV consists of a external membrane that is derived from the host cell, a protein core (p17 matrix, p24 capsid, p7 nucleocapsid) encoded by *gag* genes, and a diploid genome with two copies of the viral RNA genome and the reverse transcriptase, ribonuclease, and protease encoded by the *pol* gene within the core. In addition, HIV possesses two important envelope proteins encoded by the *env* gene: **gp41 and gp120**.

II. NEUTROPENIC AND HIV PATIENTS

A. Bacteria

Listeria monocytogenes

- Facultative-intracellular gram-positive bacillus
- Catalase +
- Facultative anaerobe

HARDCORE

ELISA is the primary screening test to detect HIV. **Western blot** is the confirming test. **PCR and viral load tests** allow monitoring of drug effect on viral load.

HARDCORE

Current principles of HIV therapy (remember, *there is no cure for HIV*):

1. Recommendations for initiating therapy:
   - Symptomatic HIV (e.g., presence of opportunistic infections).
   - Asymptomatic HIV patients with <200 CD4 cells/μL.
   - Asymptomatic HIV patients with >200 CD4 cells/μL may also start therapy depending on their total CD4 count and rate of decline, as well as the HIV RNA level in their plasma.

2. All HIV therapy should consist of at least a **three-drug regimen**.

3. Classes of anti-HIV drugs include:
   - Nucleoside, nucleotide, and non-nucleoside inhibitors (NRTI, NtRTIs, and NNRTI) of the viral enzyme **reverse transcriptase**.
   - Inhibitors of the viral **protease enzyme** (protease inhibitors or PIs).
   - Inhibitors of **viral entry** into CD4 cells.

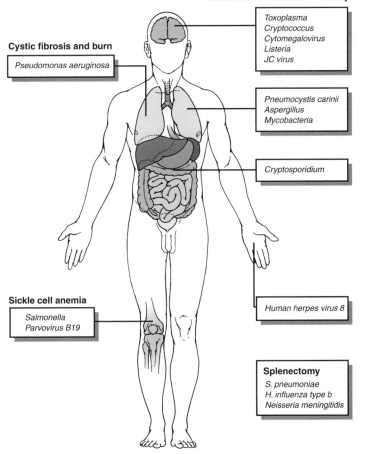

Figure 9–1 Overview of infections in immunocompromised patients.

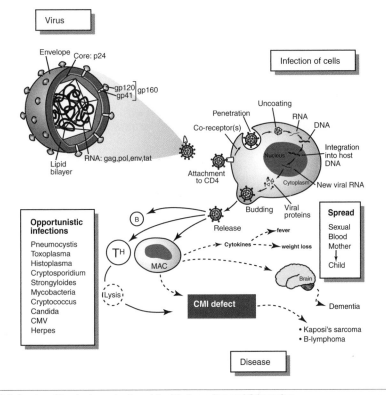

Figure 9–2 Overview of the structure and pathogenicity of the human immunodeficiency virus.

CLINICAL CORRELATES—MENINGITIS

➤ *Listeria* meningitis is the *most commonly occurring meningitis in immunocompromised patients*. This organism grows well in a refrigerated environment and is classically transmitted by *ingesting contaminated cheese*. Once in the bloodstream, *Listeria* has a predilection for the central nervous system (as well as the placenta).

  ▪ **Remember: LISteria LIves in LIndberger cheese!** (or any kind of cheese)

➤ *Listeria* is a facultative-intracellular organism that *reorganizes host cell actin*, resulting in "actin trails" that propel *Listeria* directly into other cells without exposure to the extracellular environment.

➤ Laboratory identification consists of isolating the organism on blood agar (*beta-hemolytic*) as well as identifying *Listeria*'s characteristic *"tumbling motility"* in 25°C broth cultures.

B. Mycobacterium

Mycobacterium tuberculosis

- Acid-fast rod
- Catalase +
- Aerobic

CLINICAL CORRELATES—TUBERCULOSIS

➤ Tuberculosis(TB) infection is the leading cause of death worldwide, but within developed countries TB infections are most commonly seen in the immunocompromised population (specifically HIV+).

➤ *M. tuberculosis* transmission occurs by the *inhalation of the tubercle bacillus*. After reaching the alveolar space, the tubercle bacilli proliferate, activating macrophages and sensitizing T-cells that result in the formation of *nodular granulomatous structures*. Bacilli proliferate until the host mounts a *cell-mediated immune response* (within 2 to 6 weeks after infection), resulting in the formation of *caseating necrosis* at the center of the granuloma that contains viable mycobacteria. Eventually, bacilli enter local lymph nodes, resulting in *lymphadenopathy*.

➤ Clinical findings are typically insignificant during primary TB infection. After the primary infection, M. *tuberculosis* may remain latent within the host. However, if the host immune system is compromised, a reactivation of a primary infection can occur *localizing in the lung apices*. Symptoms include cough with bloody sputum, night sweats, fever, anorexia, and weight loss. *Most patients with clinically relevant TB are diagnosed during the secondary reactivation of the primary infection*.

Mycobacterium avium-intracellulare

- Acid-fast rod
- Catalase +
- Intracellular
- Aerobic

CLINICAL CORRELATES—MYCOBACTERIUM AVIUM COMPLEX (MAC)

➤ MAC infection (which consists of one or both M. *avium* and M. *intracellulare*) in the HIV patient results in fever, night sweats, diarrhea, and focal inflammatory lymphadenitis. The risk of MAC in patients with HIV infection significantly increases as the *CD4 cell number declines below 50 cells/mm³*. These patients should be prophylactically placed on either *clarithromycin or azithromycin*.

C. Fungi

Aspergillus

- Ubiquitous filamentous fungus
- Airborne spores (conidia)

CLINICAL CORRELATES—PULMONARY ASPERGILLOSIS, ASPERGILLOMA, DISSEMINATED DISEASE INVOLVING THE CENTRAL NERVOUS SYSTEM, HEART, KIDNEY, AND SINUSES

➤ Pulmonary involvement is the most common presentation of aspergillosis in the neutropenic or HIV-infected patient. Pulmonary aspergillosis is characterized by an *upper lung lobe cavitary lesion*, focal alveolar infiltrates, fever, and cough.

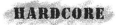

HARDCORE

Listeria enters cells by *binding to E-cadherin on the host cell*, enabling it to spread from cell to cell without exposure to the extracellular environment.

HARDCORE

The tuberculosis lesion (which typically occurs subpleurally along lung fissure lines) is produced by the expansion of the tubercle into the lung parenchyma, along with lymph node involvement, and is called the **Ghon complex**.

HARDCORE

Mycolic acid is the major constituent of the mycobacterium cell envelope and confers the ability of resisting destaining by acid alcohol after staining by aniline dyes, leading to the term *acid-fast bacillus (AFB)*. Remember that all mycobacteria are "acid-fast," and thus term *acid-fast bacilli (AFB)* is essentially synonymous with mycobacteria. *Mycobacterium* specimens may also be stained with the *Ziehl-Neelsen stain*.

HARDCORE

TB infections can be associated with inner city populations, injection drug users, and prison populations.

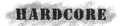

HARDCORE

TB is capable of spreading hematogenously to produce disseminated TB with lesions in many organs and a high mortality rate. **Miliary TB** refers to disseminated disease with organ lesions that resemble millet seeds.

➤ In the immunocompromised patient, the presence of a cavitary lesion (typically from previous TB infection) can lead to the development of a *fungus ball, or aspergilloma*. Typically, this develops within the parenchyma of the lung, but can occur in other organs such as the kidney or brain.

Cryptococcus neoformans

- Yeast form only

CLINICAL CORRELATES—CRYPTOCOCCAL MENINGOENCEPHALITIS AND CRYPTOCOCCAL PNEUMONIA

➤ Cryptococcal infection is common in the general population, but within the immuno-competant person it typically results in a subclinical, asymptomatic infection. When *Cryptococcus* infection occurs in the immunocompromised host (occurring in *HIV patients with cell counts less than 100/µL*) it can be fatal.

➤ *Cryptococcus* is found in *pigeon droppings*.

➤ *Cryptococcal meningoencephalitis* is a serious infection that may result in coma or death and presents with symptoms of stiff neck, photophobia, malaise, and fever. Diagnosis is made by obtaining CSF fluid with lumbar puncture. The polysaccharide capsules surrounding C. *neoformans* are visualized with *India ink* under the microscope.

➤ *Cryptococcal pneumonia* presents with vague symptoms of fever, cough, and dyspnea and diagnosis requires a sputum sample for culture and histology.

Pneumocystis carinii

- Fungus/protozoan

CLINICAL CORRELATES—PNEUMOCYSTIS PNEUMONIA

➤ Pulmonary *P. carinii* (PCP) infections occur most commonly in the HIV-afflicted immunocompromised population and presents with marked hypoxemia, dyspnea, cough, and bilateral interstitial lung infiltrates on chest X-ray. Standard of care for HIV patients requires placing them on *PCP prophylaxis with oral trimethoprim-sulfamethoxazole* (TMP-SMX) when their *CD4 count is less than 200/mm*. Patients not receiving prophylaxis are nine times more likely to develop PCP within 6 months.

D. Parasites

Cryptosporidium

- Protozoa
- Obligate intracellular parasite
- Oocyst

CLINICAL CORRELATES—CRYPTOSPORIDIOSIS (DIARRHEA)

➤ *Cryptosporidium* infection presents as acute, watery, and nonbloody diarrhea in immunocompromised patients. This bug is transmitted in *undercooked meat*.

➤ Diagnosis of *Cryptosporidium* is made by acid-fast staining of stool to detect oocyts.

Toxoplasma gondii

- Protozoa
- Obligate intracellular parasite
- Trophozoites
- Oocyst

CLINICAL CORRELATES—CNS MASS LESIONS

➤ Toxoplasmosis is a blood protozoan acquired from the ingestion of *undercooked or raw meat*. In immunocompromised patients, this infection can lead to CNS sequelae characterized by *round mass lesions with ring enhancement on head MRI*.

E. Viruses

Cytomegalovirus (CMV)

- Double-stranded DNA
- Herpesvirus
- Icosahedral nucleocapsid

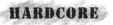

Intact neutrophil and macrophage function are the most important factors for successful host defense against *Aspergillus* infection.

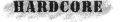

PCP is diagnosed from sputum samples that appear like a *flying saucer with silver staining*.

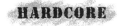

It is currently not known if PCP is a fungus or protozoan.

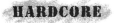

The immediate host of *T. gondii* is the cat, so this infection is also transmitted via *cat feces*.

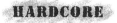

CMV pneumonia is characterized by *intracellular inclusion bodies*.

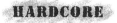

There may be a link between CMV infection and the development of atherosclerosis.

CLINICAL CORRELATES—PNEUMONITIS, CHORIORETINITIS

➤ CMV pneumonitis and retinitis are typically seen in bone or lung transplantation and in HIV patients. Primary CMV infection occurs through *interpersonal or sexual contact*, or by direct inoculation with infected cells or body fluids.

Human Herpesvirus 8

- Double-stranded DNA
- Gamma herpesvirus
- Icosahedral nucleocapsid

CLINICAL CORRELATES—KAPOSI'S SARCOMA

➤ Kaposi's sarcoma is a low-grade vascular tumor associated with the coinfection of human herpesvirus 8 (HHV-8) in AIDS patients. Human herpesvirus 8 (HHV-8) is a *lymphotropic virus* that increases cell proliferation and contributes to the formation of malignancies via an *envelope glycoprotein B (gB)* that binds cells and initiates cellular adhesion.

JC Virus

- Papovavirus

CLINICAL CORRELATES—PROGRESSIVE MULTIFOCAL LEUKOENCEPHALOPATHY

➤ JC virus is characterized by a rare CNS disease that causes *demyelination* by infecting and killing oligodendrocytes. This disease only occurs in patients with impaired immune function.

➤ JC virus is spread by respiratory droplets and contact with infected urine.

III. SPLEEN-DEFICIENT PATIENTS

The spleen consists of a series of sinusoids that filter blood and sequester senescent, rigid erythrocytes from circulation. The spleen also contains mononuclear phagocytes that remove and ingest circulating bacteria, and is the largest lymphoid organ within the body, containing almost half of the total immunoglobulin-producing B-lymphocytes. Thus, the immunologic function of the spleen is to:

1. *Clear bacteria from circulation*.
2. Process foreign material, stimulating *production of opsonizing antibodies*, particularly *IgM antibodies*.

Splenectomized patients or those with impaired splenic function are at risk for serious infection caused by *encapsulated pathogens* cleared normally by opsonization:

- *S. pneumoniae*
- *Haemophilus influenzae*
- *Neisseria meningitidis*

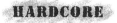

Patients who have had a splenectomy should be immunized with *S. pneumoniae*, meningococcal polysaccharide, and conjugate *H. influenzae* type b vaccine. Ideally, these vaccines should be administered 2 weeks prior to splenectomy.

IV. SICKLE-CELL PATIENTS

Sickle-cell anemia is an autosomal-dominant anemia characterized by sickle-shaped erythrocytes and accelerated hemolysis. Infection is a major cause of morbidity and mortality in these patients due to splenic dysfunction secondary to RBC sickling within the spleen and an inability of the spleen to filter microorganisms from the blood. These patients are predisposed to infection by encapsulated organisms (see above), salmonella bone infection, and parvovirus-related aplastic crisis.

A. Bacteria

Salmonella

- Gram-negative rod
- Beta-hemolytic
- Non-lactose fermenter

CLINICAL CORRELATES—OSTEOMYELITIS

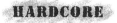

Osteomyelitis in sickle-cell patients primarily affects long bones (the femur, tibia, fibula and humerus).

➤ Sickle-cell patients are at an increased risk of osteomyelitis due to the higher rates of bone infarction in this population. The most commonly associated organism causing osteomyelitis in this population is the *Salmonella* species. *Staphylococcus aureus*, the most common etiologic agent in patients without sickle-cell anemia, accounts for less than 25% of cases.

B. Viruses

Parvovirus B 19

- Single-stranded, DNA virus
- Parvoviridae
- Non-enveloped
- Icosahedral nucleocapsid

CLINICAL CORRELATES—APLASTIC CRISIS

➤ Parvovirus B 19 *replicates within erythroid progenitor cells* and can result in the arrest of erythropoiesis, erythroid precursor cell lysis, and the ultimate *loss of mature red blood cells*. In compromised individuals, like sickle-cell patients, *Parvovirus* infection can lead to an aplastic crisis.

V. CYSTIC FIBROSIS AND BURN VICTIMS

A. Bacteria

Pseudomonas aeruginosa

- Gram-negative rod
- Aerobe
- Oxidase +
- Non-lactose fermenter

CLINICAL CORRELATES—PNEUMONIA, RESPIRATORY FAILURE, BACTEREMIA, WOUND INFECTION

➤ *P. aeruginosa* has a predilection for cystic fibrosis and burn patients, commonly showing up on board exams in these patient populations. *P. aeruginosa* is the most common cause of *respiratory failure in patients with cystic fibrosis* and is responsible for the death of the majority of these patients.

➤ Patients with extensive burns have reduced neutrophil activity, T-lymphocyte dysfunction, and an imbalance in cytokine production, which allows *P. aeruginosa* to *colonizatize burn sites*. This may lead to infection spread through the lymphatics, invading blood vessels and resulting in systemic bacteremia. Remember that *P. aeruginosa* forms *blue-green—colored colonies* when cultured.

HARDCORE REVIEW TABLES—MICROBIOLOGY IN IMMUNOCOMPROMISED PATIENTS (TABLE 9-1 TO TABLE 9-4)

TABLE 9-1	Neutropenic and HIV Patients		
BUGS	**BUG POINTS**	**MOST COMMON PRESENTATION**	**HARDCORE MICROBIOLOGY**
Bacteria			
Listeria	• Facultative-intracellular gram-positive bacillius • Catalase + • Facultative anaerobe	Meningitis	Transmitted by ingesting contaminated cheese
Mycobacterium			
Mycobacterium tuberculosis	• Acid-fast rod • Catalase + • Aerobic	Tuberculosis	Immunocompromised at risk, reactivation of primary disease occurs in lung apices, caseating necrosis, ghon complex, and nodular granulomas
Mycobacterium avium/ intracellulare	• Acid-fast rod • Catalase + • Intracellular • Aerobic	MAC	HIV patients with CD4 count <50

(Continued)

TABLE 9-1	Neutropenic and HIV Patients (cont.)		
BUGS	**BUG POINTS**	**MOST COMMON PRESENTATION**	**HARDCORE MICROBIOLOGY**
Fungi			
Aspergillus	• Ubiquitous filamentous fungus • Airborne spores (conidia)	Pulmonary aspergillosis, aspergilloma	Can form a cavitary lesion leading to the development of a fungus ball
Cryptococcus neoformans	• Yeast form only	Cryptococcal pneumonia, meningoencephalitis	Found in pigeon droppings; India-ink stain testing
Pneumocystis carinii (PCP)	• Fungus/protozoan	Pneumocystis pneumonia	Flying saucer appearing with silver stain; AIDS patients with CD4 count <200 at risk
Parasites			
Cryptosporidium	• Protozoa • Obligate intracellular parasite • Oocyst	Cryptosporidiosis (diarrhea)	Fecal–oral transmission, common in daycare setting
Toxoplasma gondii	• Protozoa • Obligate intracellular parasite • Trophozoites • Oocyst	CNS mass lesions	Spread in under-cooked meat and cat feces (changing the litter)
Virus			
Cytomegalovirus	• Double-stranded DNA • Herpesvirus • Icosahedral nucleocapsid	CMV pneumonitis, chorioretinitis	Replicates in fibroblasts
Human herpes virus 8	• Double-stranded DNA • Gamma herpesvirus • Icosahedral nucleocapsid • Papovavirus	Kaposi's sarcoma	Linked to B-cell lymphomas and multiple myeloma in certain patients
JC virus		Progressive multifocal leukoencephalopathy	Causes demyelination by infecting and killing oligodendrocytes

TABLE 9-2	Spleen Deficient (Encapsulated Organisms)		
BUGS	**BUG POINTS**	**MOST COMMON PRESENTATION**	**HARDCORE MICROBIOLOGY**
Bacteria			
Streptococcus pneumoniae	• Gram-positive • Alpha-hemolytic • Ferments inulin • Facultative anaerobe	Sepsis	Alpha-hemolysis on blood agar, part of normal oropharyngeal flora
Haemophilus influenzae	• Gram-negative rod • Aerobe • Oxidase + • Non-lactose fermenter	Sepsis	Cultured on blood agar, not airborne
Neisseria meningitidis	• Gram-negative diplococci • Ferments maltose and glucose • Oxidase + • Anaerobe	Sepsis	Kidney bean shape

TABLE 9-3	Sickle-Cell Patients		
BUGS	**BUG POINTS**	**MOST COMMON PRESENTATION**	**HARDCORE MICROBIOLOGY**
Bacteria			
Salmonella	• Gram-negative rod • Beta-hemolytic • Non-lactose fermenter	Osteomyelitis	Wide host range (more than human)
Virus			
Parvovirus **B 19**	• Single-stranded, DNA virus • Parvoviridae • Non-enveloped • Icosahedral nucleocapsid	Aplastic crisis	Replicates within erythroid progenitor cells

TABLE 9-4 Cystic Fibrosis and Burn Victims

Bugs	Bug Points	Most Common Presentation	Hardcore Microbiology
Pseudomonas aeruginosa	• Gram-negative rod • Aerobe • Oxidase + • Non-lactose fermenter	Pneumonia, respiratory failure, bacteremia, wound infection	Opportunistic pathogen, produces blue and green pigments when cultured

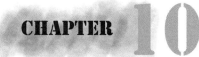
Infections of the Sexually Active

The population of sexually active individuals is a unique demographic group that aquires a very specific subset of infections on the USMLE examination. Be sure you understand how to differentiate these organisms clinically and in the laboratory.

Bugs discussed in this chapter:

- Human Papillomavirus
- Molluscum contagiosum virus
- *Calymmatobacterium granulomatis*
- *Haemophilus ducreyi*
- *Chlamydia trachomatis*
- *Neisseria gonorrhoeae*
- *Treponema pallidum*

- *Ureaplasma urealyticum*
- Hepatitis B (HBV)
- Hepatitis D (HDV)
- *Trichomonas vaginalis*
- *Gardnerella vaginalis*
- Herpes simplex virus
- *Sarcoptes scabiei*

I. BACTERIA

Calymmatobacterium granulomatis

CLINICAL CORRELATES—GRANULOMA INGUINALE

➤ Granuloma inguinale has *nonpainful*, raised red ulcerated lesions with rolled, raised edges that have a "*beefy red appearance.*" These lesions are *highly vascular* and bleed with contact.

Chlamydia trachomatis

- Gram-negative
- Obligate intracellular parasite

CLINICAL CORRELATES—NONGONOCOCCAL URETHRITIS (MEN), PELVIC INFLAMMATORY DISEASE (WOMEN), LYMPHOGRANULOMA VENEREUM

➤ *C. trachomatis* is the *most common sexually transmitted disease caused by a bacterium*, resulting in nongonococcal urethritis in men and pelvic inflammatory disease (PID) in women. Women with PID present with pain, adnexal tenderness, and the so-called **chandelier sign**, referring to the patient's immediate reaction to the exquisite pain associated with cervical motion (use your imagination). Untreated PID can lead to infertility or ectopic pregnancy.

➤ *C. trachomatis* is also responsible for causing genital ulcers called **lymphogranuloma venereum** (LGV). It results from *C. trachomatis*-induced lymphoproliferative reaction and consists of three types of serovars: L1, L2, and L3.

➤ *C. trachomatis* uses adhesions to attach to cell membranes, replicates in phagocytic vesicles in the host cell, and eventually results in cell death. Diagnosis includes *cytoplasmic inclusions seen on Giemsa stain*.

Gardnerella vaginalis

- Gram-negative rod

CLINICAL CORRELATES—BACTERIAL VAGINITIS

➤ Bacterial vaginosis (BV) is the most common cause of vaginitis in women prior to menopause. A patient with bacterial vaginosis typically presents with a "*fishy*" *vaginal discharge* that may involve irritative symptoms. Although sexual activity is not required to acquire bacterial vaginosis, sexual activity increases the risk of BV infection.

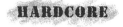

HARDCORE

Lymphogranuloma venereum infection is found in tropical and subtropical areas of the world.

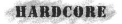

HARDCORE

In addition to *Yersinia pestis* (plague), *C. trachomatis* associated LGV is also associated with the formation of fluctuant **buboes** (lymphoid regions with exquisite tenderness, erythema, and edema of the overlying skin).

HARDCORE

Severe *C. trachomatis* infection may be associated with perihepatitis, or **Fitz-Hugh-Curtis syndrome**, in which inflammation leads to fibrosis and scarring of the anterior surface of the liver and peritoneum.

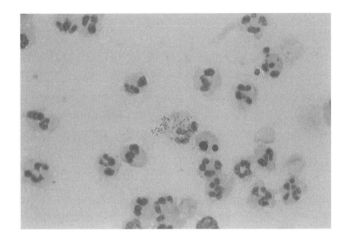

Figure 10–1 Gram stain of *Neisseria gonorrhoeae* in urethral exudate. *(Reprinted with permission from McClatchey KD. Clinical Laboratory Medicine, 2nd Edition. Philadelphia: Lippincott Williams & Wilkins, 2002:F51.4).*

➤ Diganosis includes microscopic inspection for **clue cells**, which are vaginal epithelial cells covered with bacteria that appear "blurry" when viewed under the microscope.

Haemophilus ducreyi

- Gram-negative rod

CLINICAL CORRELATES—CHANCROID

➤ *H. ducreyi* infection results in chancroid formation, which are erythematous papules that evolve into *very painful ulcers* with gray and yellow purulent exudates.

➤ *H. ducreyi* has a *"school of fish"* appearance under the microscope.

Neisseria gonorrhoeae

- Gram-negative diplococci
- Ferments only glucose
- Oxidase +
- Anaerobe

CLINICAL CORRELATES—GONORRHEA, GONOCOCCAL URETHRITIS (MEN), PELVIC INFLAMMATORY DISEASE AND SALPINGITIS (WOMEN)

➤ Gonorrhea is a sexually transmitted disease characterized by urethra purulent discharge and pain during urination. In women, this infection is typically localized to the urethra or endocervix, but can progress to involve the uterus and fallopian tubes resulting in pelvic inflammatory disease or salpingitis.

➤ *N. gonorrhoeae* contains *pili and membrane proteins* that allow attachment to host cell surfaces.

➤ Diagnosis is made by culture of the discharge revealing *pairs of kidney-shaped diplococci within PMNs* (Fig. 10-1).

Treponema pallidum

- Gram-negative, corkscrew shaped
- Spirochete

CLINICAL CORRELATES —SYPHILIS, CONDYLOMATA LATA

➤ Syphilis is a sexually transmitted disease that occurs in three distinct stages.

- *Stage 1*—After contact with an infectious lesion, a *painless* (versus the *painful* chancre of H. ducreyi), indurated ulcer, or **chancre**, develops. This lasts for 3 to 8 weeks.
- *Stage 2*—This lesion eventually disappears, and within 3 months the second stage of disease develops. The second stage includes systemic symptoms, a rash *that involves the hands and feet*, and *condylomata lata*, which are painless, moist, nonindurated lesions with high concentrations of *Treponema*. This stage is highly infective.
- *Stage 3*—The final, or tertiary stage of untreated syphilis infection occurs after a period of latency from clinical symptoms following resolution of secondary syphilis symptoms. Tertiary syphilis is characterized by *degenerative changes in the CNS*, cardiovascular complications, degeneration of the knee joint (Charcot's joint), and granulomatous lesions called *gummas*, on the skin, bones, and liver.

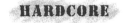

Bacterial vaginosis results from a change in the vaginal flora characterized by a reduction in lactobacilli and an increase in the prevalence of several species including *Gardnerella vaginalis, Mycoplasma hominis*, and anaerobic gram-negative rods.

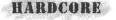

Gonococcal bacteremia may result in the formation of hemorrhagic papules and pustules on the skin, tenosynovitis, and suppurative arthritis (septic arthritis) that is usually seen in the knees, ankles, and wrists. However, only 30% of these patients will have positive gonococci cultures from synovial fluid or blood.

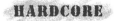

Darkfield microscopy is used for direct visualization during the primary stage of syphilis. Serological testing includes the primary *VDRL/RPR nontreponemal test* (nonspecific) and the secondary *FTA-ABS* (specific).

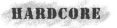

A positive FTA-ABS for syphilis can remain positive for the remainder of the patient's lifetime.

Ureaplasma urealyticum

- Pleomorphic
- No cell wall
- Urease +

CLINICAL CORRELATES—NONGONOCOCCAL URETHRITIS AND CHORIOAMNIONITIS

➤ *U. urealyticum* is a sexually transmitted disease with a predilection for having a **high colonization rate in men**, resulting in urethritis. *U. urealyticum* can also cause infection of the amniotic fluid, membranes, placenta, and uterus (chorioamnionitis) in pregnant women.

II. VIRUSES

Herpes Simplex Virus

- Double-stranded, linear DNA virus
- *Herpesviridae*

CLINICAL CORRELATES—GENITAL HERPES

➤ Herpes simplex virus consists of two serotypes, HSV-1 and HSV-2, with **HSV-2** responsible for 85% of genital infections. Infection begins with mild paresthesia and burning and is followed by vesicular lesions characterized by shallow ulcers and a red border.

Human Papillomavirus (HPV)

- *Papovaviridae*
- Double-stranded, circular DNA virus

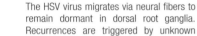

The HSV virus migrates via neural fibers to remain dormant in dorsal root ganglia. Recurrences are triggered by unknown causes and occur in 30% of patients.

CLINICAL CORRELATES—CONDYLOMATA ACUMINATA (GENITAL WARTS), CERVICAL CANCER

➤ Human papillomavirus (HPV) infects epithelial tissues and mucous membranes and is responsible for condylomata acuminata, or **genital warts**. Condylomata acuminata are dry, friable, "**cauliflower-like**" lesions found on the genital or anal region and are transmitted via sexual contact. Common types of HPV resulting in condylomata infection include 6 and 11.

➤ In women, HPV infection may include cervical lesions (including cervical intraepithelial neoplasia). **High-risk HPV types 16 and 18** are more frequently isolated in cervical cancer tissue than other types. Cervical infection by HPV is the **most common cause of cervical malignancy** and can progress to cervical intraepithelial neoplasia or carcinoma within 2 to 3 years if left untreated.

Molluscum Contagiosum Virus

- Double-stranded, DNA virus
- Poxvirus

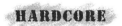

The Papanicolaou (Pap) smear is the cytologic technique used to detect HPV disease of the cervix and vagina, and is typically performed annually in sexually active women.

CLINICAL CORRELATES—GENITAL MOLLUSCUM CONTAGIOSUM

➤ The lesions of genital molluscum contagiosum consist of a **raised papule with a waxy core and central indentation**. These lesions can be removed with cryotherapy.

Hepatitis B (HBV)

- Double-stranded, circular DNA virus
- *Hepadnavirus*

CLINICAL CORRELATES—ACUTE AND CHRONIC HEPATITIS, HEPATOCELLULAR CARCINOMA

➤ Hepatitis B is a big, enveloped, and extremely contagious virus that lives in human body fluids including **semen, blood, urine, saliva, and breast milk**. Transmission takes place through the exchange of bodily fluids, typically through **sexual contact, needle-sharing**, or accidental medical exposure including needle sticks and blood spray on mucus membranes.

➤ HBV causes acute and chronic hepatitis that may evolve into fulminant hepatitis (2% mortality) and cirrhosis with portal hypertension. In addition, HBV's DNA can incorporate into hepatocyte DNA and cause malignant transformation. This **increases the risk of developing** *primary hepatocellular carcinoma up to 200 times that of a non-HBV carrier.* Serologic diagnosis of HBV infection is a Step 1 favorite.

➤ The intact HBV virus is called a **Dane particle** and its DNA codes for three surface proteins, all of which act as antigens to the human immune system (See chapter 17):

1. **Surface antigen (HBsAg)**—Presence of surface antigen *indicates active infection*. Serologically, this is the initial marker of infection and will be seen in blood tests for the first 6 months of infection.

2. **Core antigen (HBcAg)**.

3. **Pre-core protein (HBeAg)**—Presence of pre-core protein indicates *high infectious capability and active disease*. These antigens can be serologically identified after the second month of infection.

   ▪ Remember: H*Be*AG = *Be*ware, pre-core protein means highly infectious

   • As with any antigen, the human immune system forms antibodies to these foreign invaders. Serologic tests for both HBV antigens and the following formed antibodies identify the state of HBV infection:

   ▪ **Anti-HBsAg**—Antibodies to surface antigen indicate *immunity to HBV. People vaccinated against HBV will possess these antibodies*. Antibodies to HBsAg are seen after the sixth month of infection.

   ▪ **IgM anti-HBcAg**—Indicates a *new* infection.

   ▪ **IgG anti-HBcAg**—Indicates an *old* infection.

   ▪ **Anti-HBeAg**—Antibodies to pre-core proteins still indicate an infectious state, but less so than those with pre-core protein *antigens* (HBeAg). These antibodies will be seen serologically soon after the presence of HBeAg (end of the first month).

Hepatitis D (HDV)

• Single-stranded, circular RNA virus (incomplete)
• Helical nucleocapsid

CLINICAL CORRELATES—HEPATITIS

➤ The hepatitis D virus requires the presence of the hepatitis B virus (HBV) for complete virion assembly and secretion, and therefore is unable to cause infection without the coexistence of simultaneous hepatitis B infection.

III. PARASITES

Sarcoptes scabiei

• Ectoparasite

CLINICAL CORRELATES—SCABIES

➤ Scabies is caused by S. *scabiei*, or itch mites, which burrow, reproduce, and reside in human skin. Scabies infection presents as erythematous papules and vesicles in the genital region, as well as in interdigital web spaces, anterior axillary folds, and periumbilical skin.

Trichomonas vaginalis

• Flagellated protozoan

CLINICAL CORRELATES—TRICHOMONAL VAGINITIS

➤ Trichomonal vaginitis is a common sexually transmitted disease in women and presents with *frothy discharge with a fishy odor*, pruritus, and dysuria.

➤ The presence of *pear-shaped, motile trichomonads on wet mount* is diagnostic of infection. Culture on *Diamond's medium* has a high sensitivity and specificity for this infection.

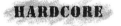

Because of the dependence of HDV on HBV, the diagnosis of hepatitis D cannot be made in the absence of markers of HBV infection including HBsAg or IgM antibody to hepatitis B core antigen.

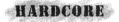

In trichomoniasis infection, punctate hemorrhages may be seen on the vaginal wall or cervix, leading to the term, "strawberry cervix."

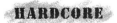

Carriage of *Trichomonas* in men is asymptomatic, self-limited, and transient.

HARDCORE REVIEW TABLES—INFECTIONS OF THE SEXUALLY ACTIVE (TABLE 10-1 TO TABLE 10-3)

TABLE 10-1 Bacteria

BUGS	BUG POINTS	MOST COMMON PRESENTATION	HARDCORE MICROBIOLOGY
Calymmatobacterium granulomatis	• Raised ulcerated lesions	Granuloma inguinale	Nonpainful, beefy red appearance
Chlamydia trachomatis	• Gram-negative • Obligate intracellular parasite	Nongonococcal urethritis (men), pelvic inflammatory disease (women), lymphogranuloma venereum	adhesions attach to cell membranes, the most common bacterial caused sexually transmitted disease, "chandelier sign" associated with cervical manipulation in patients with pelvic inflammatory disease
Gardnerella vaginalis	• Gram-negative rod	Bacterial vaginosis, vaginitis	"Fishy" vaginal discharge, "clue cells" under microscope
Haemophilus ducreyi	• Gram-negative rod	Chancroid, ulcers	Very painful, school of "fish" appearance
Neisseria gonorrhoeae	• Gram-negative diplococci • Ferments only glucose • Oxidase + • Anaerobe	Gonorrhea, gonococcal urethritis (men), pelvic inflammatory disease and salpingitis (women)	Pili and membrane proteins that allow attachment, diagnosis made by culture of discharge revealing pairs of kidney-shaped diplococci within PMNs
Treponema pallidum	• Gram-negative, corkscrew shaped • Spirochete	Syphilis, condylomata lata	Three stages: ○ *Stage 1*—painless ulcer, or "chancre," develops ○ *Stage 2*—systemic symptoms including a rash that involves the hands and feet, and condylomata lata; this stage is highly infective ○ *Stage 3*—characterized by degenerative changes in the CNS, cardiovascular complications, degeneration of the knee joint (Charcot's joint), gummas, and lesions on the skin, bones, and liver
Ureaplasma urealyticum	• Pleomorphic • No cell wall • Urease +	Nongonococcal urethritis	High colonization rate in men, resulting in urethritis

TABLE 10-2 Viruses

BUGS	BUG POINTS	MOST COMMON PRESENTATION	HARDCORE MICROBIOLOGY
Herpes simplex virus	• Double-stranded, linear DNA virus • *Herpesviridae*	Genital herpes	HSV-2 is responsible for 85% of genital infections
Human *Papillomavirus*	• Double-stranded, circular DNA virus • *Papovaviridae*	Condylomata acuminata (genital warts), cervical cancer	Replicates in the nucleus, condylomata acuminate are dry, friable, "cauliflower-like" lesions, HPV is the most common cause of cervical malignancy (types 16 and 18)
Hepatitis B	• Double-stranded, circular DNA virus • *Hepadnavirus*	Acute and chronic hepatitis, hepatocellular carcinoma	Acquired by bodily fluid exchange (sexual contact), increases risk of developing primary hepatocellular carcinoma by 200 times Serology: ○ HBsAg—infection ○ HBeAg—high infectivity ○ Anti-HBsAg—immunity
Hepatitis D	• Single-stranded, circular RNA virus (incomplete) • Helical nucleocapsid	Hepatitis	Requires the presence of the hepatitis B virus
Molluscum contagiosum virus	• Double-stranded, DNA virus • Poxvirus	Genital molluscum contagiosum	Raised papule with a waxy core and central indentation

TABLE 10-3 Parasites

BUGS	BUG POINTS	MOST COMMON PRESENTATION	HARDCORE MICROBIOLOGY
Sarcoptes scabiei	• Ectoparasite	Scabies	Burrow, reproduce, and reside in human skin
Trichomoniasis vaginalis	• Flagellated protozoan	Trichomonal vaginitis	Presents with frothy discharge with a fishy odor, presence of strawberry cervix, motile trichomonads on wet mount is diagnostic of infection

CHAPTER 11

Infections in the Chemically Dependent

Patients inebriated by chemical substances are at an increased risk of infection by certain organisms. These organisms can gain access to tissues by aspiration of gastric contents (due to a patient's lowered level of consciousness), or by direct inoculation of organisms into the bloodstream via contaminated needles. Be on the lookout for these organisms in patients who are chemically dependent.

Bugs discussed in this chapter:

- Human immunodeficiency virus
- *Staphylococcus aureus*
- *Streptococcus pneumoniae*
- *Klebsiella pneumoniae*

- *Fusobacterium*
- *Eikenella corrodens*
- Hepatitis C
- *Pseudomonas aeruginosa*

I. IMMUNE SYSTEM

Human Immunodeficiency Virus

- Retrovirus
- Lentivirus
- Glycoproteins gp120/gp41
- Protein core encoded by gag genes

CLINICAL CORRELATES—AIDS, OPPORTUNISTIC INFECTIONS

➤ HIV is a retrovirus most commonly spread from human to human by the sharing of contaminated needles or unprotected sexual activities.

➤ Symptoms of an acute HIV infection are nonspecific and include fatigue, rash, headache, nausea, and night sweats that resolve over a few weeks. Over time, the HIV infection results in the unrelenting and extensive destruction of host CD4 cells, eventually allowing opportunistic pathogens to invade the immunocompromised host and cause disease (see Chapter 9). The more serious symptoms of opportunistic infection are often preceded by a prodrome that includes fatigue, weight loss, fever, chronic diarrhea, oral candidiasis, and lymphadenopathy.

➤ Patients involved in risky behaviors should be screened for HIV. *ELISA* is used as the primary screening test. Any positive ELISA tests should undergo *Western blot analysis* as the confirmatory test.

II. PULMONARY SYSTEM

People under the influence of alcohol, intravenous drugs, or other substances are more prone to episodes of reduced levels of consciousness than the normal person. During these times, these people risk aspirating oropharyngeal secretions, introducing enteric bacteria into the lungs and resulting in infectious pneumonia.

A. Gram-Positive Bacteria

Staphylococcus aureus

- Gram-positive cocci (clusters)
- Catalase +

- Coagulase +
- Beta-hemolytic

CLINICAL CORRELATES—HEMATOGENOUS PNEUMONIA

➤ Right-sided tricuspid valve endocarditis is most commonly encountered in IV drug users. After seeding their heart valves, patients are at risk for *S. aureus pneumonia from bacterial embolization off of an infected heart valve*. S. *aureus* pneumonia causes rapid destruction of lung parenchyma, resulting in lung cavitations, effusions, and empyema.

Streptococcus pneumoniae

- Gram-positive lancet-shaped diplococcus in chains
- Catalase –
- Ferments inulin
- Optochin-sensitive
- Alpha-hemolytic
- Facultative anaerobe

CLINICAL CORRELATES—PNEUMONIA

➤ S. *pneumoniae* is a common cause of gram-positive pneumonia in substance abusers.

➤ Under the microscope, pneumococcus appears as *lancet-shaped gram-positive cocci in pairs*.

B. Gram-Negative Bacteria

Eikenella corrodens

- Gram-negative rod
- Oxidase +

CLINICAL CORRELATES—PNEUMONIA, PERIODONTAL DISEASE

➤ *Eikenella* is another enteric bacteria found in mixed flora infections that is also associated with oral mucosal and bowel organisms.

Fusobacterium

- Gram-negative rod
- Anaerobic

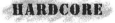

HARDCORE

Eikenella is rampant in the human mouth and may be associated with serious skin infections from *human bites*.

CLINICAL CORRELATES—PNEUMONIA, PERIODONTAL DISEASE

➤ Fusobacteria are enteric bacteria linked to *aspiration pneumonia and periodontal disease*, but can also cause abdominal abscesses and otitis media.

Klebsiella pneumoniae

- Gram-negative rod
- Lactose fermenter
- Enteric bacteria

CLINICAL CORRELATES—PNEUMONIA

➤ In debilitated patients, particularly *passed-out alcoholics* or hospitalized patients, the enteric bacteria *Klebsiella* may be aspirated from the GI tract, resulting in **bloody pneumonia**. This pneumonia is characterized by a thick sputum that, when coughed up, appears the color of *red currant jelly*.

III. CARDIOVASCULAR SYSTEM

Staphylococcus aureus

- Gram-positive cocci (clusters)
- Catalase +
- Coagulase +
- Beta-hemolytic

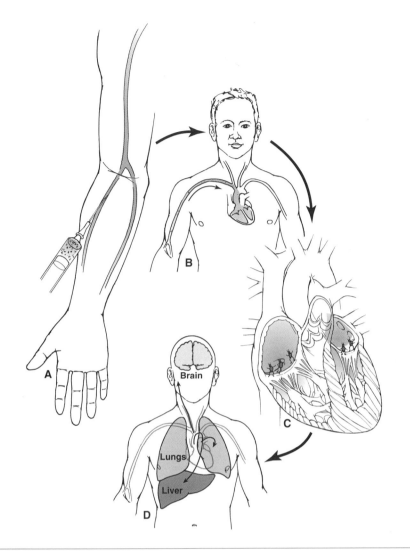

Figure 11–1 *S. aureus* endocarditis and embolization. A) a contaminated needle introduces bacteria to the normally sterile blood stream B) bacteria travel to the heart C) *S. aureus* infects heart valves causing vegetative growth D) infection may lead to metastatic foci of *S. aureus* to lungs, liver, or brain.

CLINICAL CORRELATES—ACUTE BACTERIAL ENDOCARDITIS (ABE)

➤ S. *aureus*, introduced into the bloodstream from contaminated needles, can infect normal heart valves and cause vegetative growth and valvular destruction. IV drug users classically develop *right-sided (tricuspid valve) endocarditis* from infected venous blood returning to the heart.

➤ This infection can lead to *metastatic foci* of infectious S. *aureus* to the lungs (right-sided ABE), brain (left-sided ABE), and other end organs depending on which side of the heart is infected (Fig. 11-1).

IV. GASTROINTESTINAL SYSTEM

Hepatitis B

- Double-stranded, circular DNA virus
- Hepadnavirus

CLINICAL CORRELATES—ACUTE VIRAL HEPATITIS, CHRONIC HEPATITIS, CIRRHOSIS, HEPATOCELLULAR CARCINOMA

➤ Hepatitis B virus is acquired by bodily fluid exchange. Although this typically occurs with sexual contact, hepatitis B is also transmitted from person to person by contaminated needles.

➤ The hepatitis B virion is a DNA virus that contains single-stranded breaks.

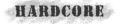

Although the most common cause of right-sided (pulmonic and tricuspid valve) endocarditis is IV drug abuse, most IV drug abuse associated endocarditis is still left-sided.

Hepatitis C

- Positive, single-stranded RNA virus
- Flavivirus

CLINICAL CORRELATES—ACUTE VIRAL HEPATITIS, CHRONIC HEPATITIS, CIRRHOSIS, HEPATOCELLULAR CARCINOMA

➤ The hepatitis C virus (HCV) is a parenterally transmitted, enveloped virus that causes acute hepatitis. Most HCV infections are persistent and chronic (80%), and typically are asymptomatic. However, 35% of patients with chronic HCV infection develop *cirrhosis, liver failure, or hepatocellular carcinoma (HCC)*.

➤ Patients with suspected HCV infection are screened for *anti-HCV antibodies*.

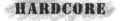

HCV infection may result in HCC after 10 to 30 years of infection. HCV is able to escape the immune system by frequent viral mutations, resulting in an immunologically distinct "quasi-species."

HARDCORE

Although both HCV and HBV are blood-borne pathogens and can both be transmitted by needle-sharing or blood transfusions, HBV is classically associated with *unprotected sexual intercourse* while HCV is classically associated with *IV drug use*.

V. MUSCULOSKELETAL SYSTEM

A. Gram-Positive Bacteria

Staphylococcus aureus

- Gram-positive cocci (clusters)
- Catalase +
- Coagulase +
- Beta-hemolytic

CLINICAL CORRELATES—OSTEOMYELITIS

➤ *S. aureus* accounts for *90% of all cases of osteomyelitis*. IV drug users are at an elevated risk of developing this bone infection both directly from infection at an intravenous injection site, or indirectly via hematogenous seeding from a contaminated needle.

B. Gram-Negative Bacteria

Pseudomonas aeruginosa

- Gram-negative rod
- Aerobe
- Oxidase +
- Non-lactose fermenter

CLINICAL CORRELATES—OSTEOMYELITIS

➤ In IV drug users, *Pseudomonas* infections may result in *vertebral body osteomyelitis*. Most commonly, patients who develop *Pseudomonas* osteomyelitis are *young males*.

HARDCORE REVIEW TABLES—INFECTIONS IN THE CHEMICALLY DEPENDENT (TABLE 11-1 TO TABLE 11-5)

TABLE 11-1 Immune System			
BUGS	**BUG POINTS**	**MOST COMMON PRESENTATION**	**HARDCORE MICROBIOLOGY**
Viruses			
Human immunodeficiency virus	• Retrovirus • Lentivirus • Glycoproteins gp120/gp41 • Protein core encoded by *gag* genes	Opportunistic infection	ELISA is used as a primary screening test, Western blot is confirmatory

TABLE 11-2 Pulmonary System

BUGS	BUG POINTS	MOST COMMON PRESENTATION	HARDCORE MICROBIOLOGY
Gram-Positive Bacteria			
Staphylococcus aureus	• Gram-positive cocci (clusters) • Catalase + • Coagulase + • Beta-hemolytic	Pneumonia	Results following right-sided tricuspid valve endocarditis, causes rapid destruction of lung parenchyma
Streptococcus pneumoniae	• Gram-positive, lancet-shaped diplococcus in chains • Catalase – • Ferments inulin • Optochin-sensitive • Alpha-hemolytic • Facultative anaerobe	Pneumonia	Lancet-shaped gram-positive diplococci arranged in pairs
Gram-Negative Bacteria			
Eikenella corrodens	• Gram-negative rod • Oxidase +	Pneumonia, periodontal disease	Also causes infections from human bites
Fusobacterium	• Gram-negative rod • Anaerobic	Pneumonia, periodontal disease	Enteric bacteria
Klebsiella pneumoniae	• Gram-negative rod • Lactose fermenter • Enteric bacteria	Pneumonia	Occurs in passed-out alcoholics, sputum appears the color of red currant jelly

TABLE 11-3 Cardiovascular System

BUGS	BUG POINTS	MOST COMMON PRESENTATION	HARDCORE MICROBIOLOGY
Gram-Positive Bacteria			
Staphylococcus aureus	• Gram-positive cocci (clusters) • Coagulase + • Catalase + • Beta-hemolytic	Acute bacterial endocarditis	Infects normal heart valves, causing vegetative growth and valvular destruction; classically right-sided

TABLE 11-4 Gastrointestinal System

BUGS	BUG POINTS	MOST COMMON PRESENTATION	HARDCORE MICROBIOLOGY
Viruses			
Hepatitis B virus	• Double-stranded, circular DNA virus • Hepadnavirus	Acute viral hepatitis, chronic hepatitis, cirrhosis, hepatocellular carcinoma	Increases risk of developing primary hepatocellular carcinoma by 200 times
Hepatitis C virus	• Positive, single-DNA virus stranded RNA virus • Flavivirus • Enveloped	Acute viral hepatitis, chronic hepatitis, cirrhosis, hepatocellular carcinoma	Majority of chronic cases are asymptomatic, screening by serology for anti-HCV antibodies

TABLE 11-5 Musculoskeletal System

BUGS	BUG POINTS	MOST COMMON PRESENTATION	HARDCORE MICROBIOLOGY
Gram-Positive Bacteria			
Staphylococcus aureus	• Gram-positive cocci (clusters) • Catalase + • Coagulase + • Beta-hemolytic	Osteomyelitis	Causes 90% of all cases of osteomyelitis, direct infection at an injection site, or indirect infection from hematogenous seeding
Gram-Negative Bacteria			
Pseudomonas aeruginosa	• Gram-negative rod • Aerobe • Oxidase + • Non-lactose fermenter	Vertebral body osteomyelitis	Occurs in young male IV drug users

CHAPTER 12

Infections of World Travelers

People traveling the world are at risk of encountering a unique and typically uncommon subset of pathogens. These organisms cause specific general infections, but are more commonly associated with gastrointestinal diseases that plague the nonhygienic or uncareful traveler. Keep these bugs in your differential when test questions include a patient who has recently traveled out of the country.

Bugs discussed in this chapter:

- Yellow fever
- Dengue viruses
- *Paracoccidioides brasiliensis*
- *Plasmodia species: P. falciparum, P. vivax, P. ovale*, and *P. malariae*

- *Salmonella*
- *Escherichia coli*
- Hepatitis A
- Noroviruses
- *Entamoeba histolytica*

I. GENERAL TRAVELER INFECTIONS

A. Bacteria

Salmonella

- Gram-negative rod
- Beta-hemolytic
- Non-lactose fermenter

CLINICAL CORRELATES—TYPHOID FEVER

➤ **Typhoidal Salmonella** (*S. typhi* or *S. paratyphi*) is endemic throughout most of sub-Saharan Africa and causes the systemic illness, typhoid fever. **Typhoid fever** is characterized by fever, abdominal tenderness, *rash (rose spots)*, hepatosplenomegaly, and eventually the development of *neuropsychiatric symptoms*.

➤ Infection occurs via direct contact with an infected individual, or indirect contact with *contaminated food or water*.

B. Parasites

Plasmodium falciparum, vivax, ovale, and *malariae*

- Protozoan

CLINICAL CORRELATES—MALARIA

➤ Although malaria is caused by four members of the *Plasmodium* species, **P. falciparum, P. vivax, P. ovale**, and **P. malariae**, the majority of malaria infection is due to either P. *falciparum* or P. *vivax*, and most malaria-associated deaths are due to P. *falciparum*.

➤ Human infection by all four *Plasmodium* species occurs by *transmission of sporozoites from a bite of an infected anopheles mosquito* (Fig. 12-1). Sporozoites travel from the salivary glands of the mosquito through the bloodstream of the human to the liver. In the liver, the organism's nuclei rapidly divide until mature *schizonts* that contain thousands of daughter *merozoites*, are formed. The liver schizonts rupture within 2 weeks, releasing thousands of merozoites into the bloodstream. These merozoites then invade red blood cells (this is called *the erythrocytic stage*). Nuclear division occurs within the RBCs, again resulting in the formation of a multinucleated schizont. The RBC then lyses, releasing merozoites that lead to an immune response causing fever, chills, and sweats.

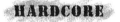

HARDCORE

P. falciparum predominates in Africa, Southeast Asia, and the Amazon basin of South America, while P. vivax is most prevalent in Central America, the Middle East, and India.

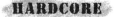

HARDCORE

Some *Plasmodium* merozoites differentiate into male or female gametocytes (sexual forms), which cause no symptoms but circulate in the bloodstream until they are ingested by a blood-feeding anopheles mosquito and complete their life-cycle within the mosquito's midgut. The sporozoites that form then migrate to the salivary glands of the mosquito, where they can reinfect humans.

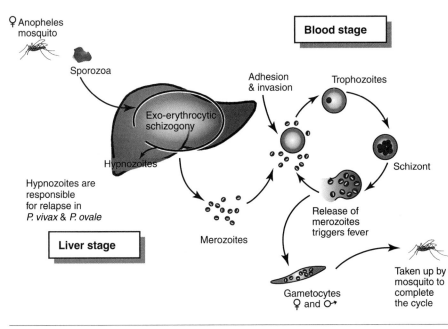

Figure 12–1 Malaria life-cycle.

➤ In *P. vivax* and *P. ovale* infections, some parasites remain dormant in the liver as *hypnozoites* and may cause relapse by reactivating after many months. Hypnozoite parasites *do not develop in P. falciparum and P. malariae* infections; thus, these organisms do not cause relapsing infections.

➤ Symptoms of malarial infections develop *only during the erythrocytic stage* of the plasmodia life cycle (Fig. 12-1).

C. Viruses

Dengue Viruses

- Positive, single-stranded RNA virus
- *Flaviviridae*
- Icosahedral symmetry
- Arbovirus

CLINICAL CORRELATES—DENGUE FEVER, DENGUE HEMORRHAGIC FEVER

➤ Dengue fever is an acute febrile illness found in tropical regions and characterized by headache, retroorbital pain, and marked muscle and joint pains, which is why the disease is sometimes called *break-bone fever*. This infection may progress into *Dengue hemorrhagic fever*, consisting of increased vascular permeability, thrombocytopenia, and hepatomegaly with abnormal liver function tests.

➤ Dengue virus is introduced by the bite of an infected mosquito and infects both humans and birds.

Yellow Fever

- Positive, single-stranded RNA virus
- *Flavaviridae*
- Icosahedral symmetry

CLINICAL CORRELATES—YELLOW FEVER

➤ Yellow fever is a mosquito-borne viral hemorrhagic fever, characterized by *jaundice*, hepatic dysfunction, renal failure, coagulopathy, hemorrhage, and shock with a high fatality rate.

➤ Yellow fever involves a primary transmission cycle that includes monkeys and *daytime-biting mosquitoes* whose larval development occurs in tree holes containing rainwater.

➤ The disease occurs in tropical regions of **South America and sub-Saharan Africa**. A safe and highly effective live, attenuated vaccine is available for travelers.

▪ Remember: **"flav"** means **yellow**, and **yellow** fever is a member of **Flaviviridae**.

D. Fungi

Paracoccidioides brasiliensis

- Dimorphic
- Conidia

CLINICAL CORRELATES—PARACOCCIDIOIDOMYCOSIS

➤ Paracoccidioidomycosis is an endemic disease found in Central and South America, and presents as **painful ulcerated lesions in the mouth**, lymphadenopathy, dysphagia, and hoarseness.

➤ Culture *P. brasiliensis* on **Sabouraud agar**.

➤ Inhalation of conidia is the route of acquisition and this fungus **affects primarily men**.

II. GASTROINTESTINAL SYSTEM

Diarrheal disease in travelers may be caused by a number of bacterial, viral, and parasitic organisms that are often transmitted by food and water. Most episodes of traveler's diarrhea occur within 4 to 14 days after arrival, and the illness is generally self-limited with symptoms lasting 1 to 5 days. Most cases of diarrhea are caused by bacteria, and the most common organism is enterotoxigenic *Escherichia coli* (ETEC).

A. Bacteria

Escherichia coli

- Gram-negative rod
- Beta-hemolytic
- Lactose fermenter
- Indole +
- Facultative anaerobe

CLINICAL CORRELATES—TRAVELER'S DIARRHEA (MONTEZUMA'S REVENGE)

➤ Enterotoxigenic *E. coli* (ETEC) is a common cause of traveler's diarrhea. ETEC survives and is transmitted in water and food supplies in the developing world. The associated diarrhea is watery and may be relatively mild or may mimic cholera. Typically the illness lasts for only 24 hours.

➤ ETEC contains two classes of secretory toxins encoded on plasmids that cause the secretion of water into the intestinal lumen and results in watery diarrhea:

▪ **Heat-labile toxins**—Act by stimulating adenylate cyclase and increasing intracellular cyclic AMP, resulting in the secretion of chloride from intestinal crypt cells and inhibition of absorption of sodium chloride at the villus tips, causing the secretion of free water (same mechanism as cholera toxin).

▪ **Heat-stable toxins**—Activate enterocyte cyclic GMP, causing the stimulation of chloride secretion and inhibition of sodium chloride absorption.

B. Viruses

Hepatitis A

- Positive, single-stranded RNA virus
- *Picornaviridae*
- Icosahedral capsid

CLINICAL CORRELATES—HEPATITIS A INFECTION

➤ Hepatitis A infection is an acute, self-limited illness spread via the **fecal–oral route** that presents with vomiting, anorexia, fever, and right upper quadrant pain. Typical symptoms of hepatitis include gastric complaints, as well as dark urine, acholic stool, jaundice,

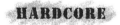

HARDCORE

E. coli also contains colonizing fimbriae that permit attachment of the bacteria to the intestine.

and pruritus. Hepatitis A can be acquired from contaminated food, usually *shellfish*, and is endemic throughout sub-Saharan Africa and in developing countries that lack adequate sanitation.

➤ Diagnosis is made by detecting anti-HAV antibodies in a patient with associated clinical presentation.

Noroviruses (Norwalk)

- Positive, single-stranded RNA virus
- *Caliciviridae*

CLINICAL CORRELATES—GASTROENTERITIS

➤ Noroviruses cause the *most common food-borne diseases and are the most frequent cause of acute gastroenteritis*. Vomiting is the predominant symptom, along with nausea and watery diarrhea. Noroviruses have been associated with large outbreaks of *diarrhea on cruise ships* and are transmitted from either the vomitus of an infected person or in aerosol form. Transmission typically occurs from a food handler via food, as well as from shellfish.

➤ The illness usually lasts for 48 to 72 hours with a rapid and full recovery.

- Remember—On your cruise to *Norway*, beware of the *Norwalk* virus causing cruise ship diarrhea.

C. Parasites

Entamoeba histolytica

- Protozoan
- Amoeba
- Oocyst

CLINICAL CORRELATES—AMEBIASIS

➤ *E. histolytica* is a parasite that represents the classic *amoeba*. About 10% of the world's population is infected with *Entamoeba*; however, most of these infections are asymptomatic.

➤ *Entamoeba* exists in two forms: *cyst and trophozoite*. The infection is spread via the fecal–oral route and follows the ingestion of cysts via contaminated food or water. Cysts pass to the small intestine, forming trophozoites. Trophozoites penetrate the mucus barrier of the colon, causing tissue destruction and increased intestinal secretion, ultimately leading to *bloody diarrhea*.

HARDCORE REVIEW TABLES—INFECTIONS OF WORLD TRAVELERS (TABLE 12-1 TO TABLE 12-4)

HARDCORE

Hepatitis A infection rarely progresses to fulminant hepatitis (1% of infections).

- Remember—Hepatitis *A* only causes *A*cute infection, but (almost) never becomes chronic.

HARDCORE

Replication of the hepatitis A virus occurs exclusively in the hepatocyte cytoplasm. Hepatocellular damage is mediated by the host's immune response, specifically via HAV-specific CD8+ T-lymphocytes and natural killer cells.

HARDCORE

Laboratory findings in symptomatic hepatitis patients are notable for marked elevations of serum aminotransferases, serum total and direct bilirubin, and alkaline phosphatase.

HARDCORE

There are no routine diagnostic assays available for noroviruses.

HARDCORE

Amebiasis may be associated with venereal transmission through fecal–oral contact in sexually active patients.

HARDCORE

Entamoeba infection may cause liver abscesses if the trophozoites enter portal blood circulation. If they penetrate the diaphragm and spread to the lung, pulmonary abscesses can result.

HARDCORE

E. histolytica's nucleus is shaped like a *bulls-eye*.

TABLE 12-1 Hardcore Malaria			
	P. FALCIPARUM	*P. VIVAX* AND *P. OVALE*	*P. MALARIAE*
Episodes of fever and chills	Usually continuous	Every 48 hours	Every 72 hours

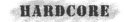

TABLE 12-2 Common Causes of Fever in Travelers
Malaria
Hepatitis
Dengue fever
Typhoid fever
Rickettsial infection
Diarrhea
Respiratory tract infections
Urinary tract infections

TABLE 12-3	General Traveler Infections		
BUGS	**BUG POINTS**	**MOST COMMON PRESENTATION**	**HARDCORE MICROBIOLOGY**
Bacteria			
Salmonella	• Gram-negative rod • Beta-hemolytic • Non-lactose fermenter	Typhoid fever • Fever • Rash (rose spots) • Hepatosplenomegaly • Neuropsychiatric symptoms	Transmission via direct contact with an infected individual or indirect contact with contaminated food or water
Parasites			
Plasmodium falciparum, vivax, ovale, malariae	• Protozoan	Malaria	Transmission of sporozoites occurs from a bite of an infected anopheline mosquito; division of the protozoan occurs within the RBCs, causing lyses, leading to an immune response causing fever, chills, and sweats; *P. falciparum* and *P. malariae* infections do not cause relapsing infections
Viruses			
Dengue viruses	• Positive, single-stranded RNA virus • *Flaviviridae* • Icosahedral symmetry • Arbovirus	Dengue fever, Dengue hemorrhagic fever • Increased vascular permeability • Thrombocytopenia • Hepatomegaly with abnormal liver function tests	Occurs via a bite of an infected mosquito, replicates in cytoplasm
Yellow fever	• Positive, single-stranded RNA virus • *Flaviviridae* • Icosahedral symmetry	Yellow fever • Hepatic dysfunction • Renal failure • Coagulopathy • Hemorrhage • Shock	From daytime-biting mosquitoes
Fungi			
Paracoccidioides brasiliensis	• Dimorphic • Conidia	Paracoccidiomycosis • Painful ulcerated lesions in the mouth	Primarily affects men, culture on Sabouraud agar

TABLE 12-4	Gastrointestinal System		
BUGS	**BUG POINTS**	**MOST COMMON PRESENTATION**	**HARDCORE MICROBIOLOGY**
Bacteria			
Escherichia coli	• Gram-negative rod • Beta-hemolytic • Lactose fermenter • Indole + • Facultative anaerobe	Traveler's diarrhea (Montezuma's revenge)	Enterotoxigenic *Escherichia coli* (ETEC) is transmitted in water and food supplies, possesses heat-labile and heat-stable toxins that increase chloride secretion and inhibit sodium chloride absorption
Viruses			
Hepatitis A	• Positive, single-stranded RNA virus • *Picornaviridae* • Icosahedral capsid	Hepatitis A infection including gastritis and transient hepatitis	Acquired typically from shellfish, can develop symptoms of hepatitis including gastric complaints, also dark urine, acholic stool, jaundice, and pruritus
Noroviruses	• Positive, single-stranded RNA virus • *Caliciviridae*	Gastroenteritis	Replicates in cytoplasm, associated with large outbreaks on cruise ships, transmitted from either the vomitus of an infected person or in aerosol form
Parasites			
Entamoeba histolytica	• Protozoan • Amoeba • Oocyst	Amebiasis • Bloody diarrhea	Ingestion of cysts by fecal-contaminated food or water, "bull's-eye" shaped nucleus

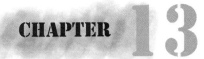

CHAPTER 13

Infections of Outdoor Enthusiasts

Several infectious organisms are commonly associated with people who enjoy spending time in the outdoors. In these question stems, people will have been hiking, camping, gardening, or around soil prior to the onset of symptoms. Be on the lookout for the following associations.

Bugs discussed in this chapter:

- *Borrelia burgdorferi*
- *Rickettsia rickettsii*
- *Sporothrix schenckii*
- *Hantavirus*
- *Histoplasma microconidia*
- *Blastomyces dermatitidis*

- *Coccidioides*
- *Clostridium tetani*
- *Naegleria fowleri*
- La Crosse (California) encephalitis virus
- *Giardia lamblia*

I. SKIN

A. Bacteria

Borrelia burgdorferi

- Gram-negative spirochete

CLINICAL CORRELATES—LYME DISEASE

➤ Lyme disease follows the transmission of the *B. burgdorferi* organism to a hiker or camper via the bite of the **Ixodes tick**. The infection initially presents with a unique skin lesion at the site of the tick bite that appears as a flat, reddened area with slowly expanding central clearing (**"bull's-eye"**), called **erythema migrans**, which is characteristic for Lyme disease. Along with a flu-like illness, fever, chills, and myalgia, this rash distinguishes the *first stage* of the disease.

➤ The *second stage* of Lyme disease occurs months after the first and consists of arthritis, meningitis, facial nerve palsy, and cardiac conduction defects. The *third stage* may begin months to years after the first stage and involves serious skin and nervous system disease, as well as joint **Lyme arthritis**.

➤ Lyme disease should be considered in any patient who presents with a rash with central clearing, flu-like symptoms, or atraumatic joint pain of unknown etiology and has recently spent times outdoors (typically in a wooded area).

➤ *Borrelia* is visualized in light microscopy using aniline dyes including Wright stain.

Rickettsia rickettsii

- Gram negative
- Obligate intracellular parasite

CLINICAL CORRELATES—ROCKY MOUNTAIN SPOTTED FEVER

➤ Rocky Mountain spotted fever is another disease transmitted via a tick bite, this time by the **Dermacentor tick** (the wood tick in the Western United States and the dog tick in the Eastern United States). *R. rickettsii* rash **begins on the ankles and wrists** and spreads both centrally and **to the palms and soles**. If untreated, the disease can cause seizures, focal neurological deficits, or gangrene of the digits, ears, and scrotum.

➤ Diagnosis of Rocky Mountain spotted fever is confirmed serologically with the **indirect fluorescent antibody (IFA) test**, and by skin biopsy.

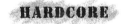

HARDCORE

Patients with a history of Lyme disease will have a false-positive VDRL (test for syphilis).

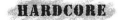

HARDCORE

The **white-footed mouse** and the **white-tailed deer** serve as reservoirs for the *B. burgdorferi* organism.

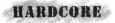

HARDCORE

The *R. rickettsii* organism is passed tick-to-tick via **transovarian transmission**.

B. Fungi

Sporothrix schenckii

- Dimorphic yeast

CLINICAL CORRELATES—SPOROTRICHOSIS

➤ Sporotrichosis is a chronic disease spread to humans when soil or moss that this fungus lives in is inoculated into human skin or subcutaneous tissue. Typically, this occurs in a healthy person who spends a lot of time outdoors planting or gardening.

➤ Infection begins as a papule at the site of inoculation, eventually becoming necrotic and ulcerating with similar lesions developing subsequently *along the lymphatic tract* proximal to the original lesion.

➤ Diagnosis is made by *culture on Sabouraud's agar.*

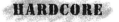

Infection with *S. schenckii* is classically seen in a *gardener whose skin has been punctured by rose thorns* contaminated with the organism.

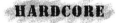

Dimorphic fungi include *Sporothrix schenckii, Candida albicans, Cryptococcus, Histoplasma, Blastomyces, Coccidioides* and *Paracoccidioides.*

II. PULMONARY SYSTEM

A. Fungi (Fig. 13-1)

Blastomyces dermatitidis

- Dimorphic fungus
- Broad-based buds
- Airborne spores

CLINICAL CORRELATES —BLASTOMYCOSIS

➤ Blastomycosis is a pulmonary pyogranulomatous infection that occurs following the *inhalation of B. dermatitidis.*

➤ The *thick cell wall* of the yeast and the glycoprotein antigen on the cell wall surface, *WI-1,* act as virulence factors. WI-1 is an adhesin that binds human macrophages and mediates yeast binding to macrophages and extracellular matrix.

Coccidioides

- Dimorphic yeast
- Endospores

CLINCAL CORRELATES—COCCIDIOIDOMYCOSIS

➤ These fungi are endemic to the *southwestern United States, as well as parts of Mexico, Central America, and South America.* Coccidioides species grow as a mold a few inches below the surface of the desert soil. Infection is acquired by inhalation of an arthroconidium, leading to the development of **Valley fever,** characterized by chest pain, cough, and fever lasting for weeks to months.

  ■ Remember: **C**occidioides lives among the **C**actuses (i.e., in the Southwest).

The *B. dermatitidis* organism is typically associated with warm, moist *soil of wooded areas* in the southeastern and south-central states that *border the Mississippi and Ohio River basins.*

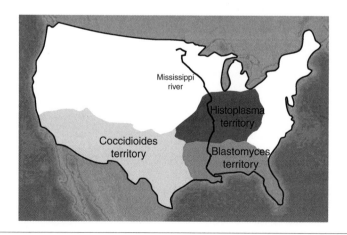

Figure 13–1 Geographic distribution of environmental fungi that cause pulmonary disease. *Coccidioides* is found in the southwestern United States, as well as parts of Mexico, Central America, and South America. *Blastomyces* is seen in southeastern and south-central states that border the Mississippi and Ohio River basins, and *Histoplasma* is located in midwestern states in the Ohio and Mississippi River valleys.

Histoplasma capsulatum

- Dimorphic yeast
- Endospores
- Facultative intracellular yeast

CLINICAL CORRELATES—HISTOPLASMOSIS

➤ Infection develops when *Histoplasma capsulatum* is inhaled into the lungs, where it germinates into yeast. Infection is most common in **midwestern states located in the Ohio and Mississippi River valleys**.

  ▪ Remember: Histoplasmosis lives in the OHio valley.

B. Viruses

Hantavirus

- Negative, single-stranded RNA virus
- Bunyavirus

CLINICAL CORRELATES—HANTAVIRUS PULMONARY SYNDROME

➤ Hanta viral infection occurs after inhaling *Hantavirus* **carried in rodent saliva or droppings**. Following an incubation period, patients develop significant hypotension with increased systemic vascular resistance and pulmonary edema. This disease has a very high mortality rate (>50%).

III. NERVOUS SYSTEM

A. Bacteria

Clostridium tetani

- Gram-positive
- Obligate anaerobe
- Spore-forming

CLINICAL CORRELATES—TETANUS

➤ *C. tetani* spores are widely present in soil. If these spores gain access to human tissue, the organism transforms into a **vegetative rod-shaped bacterium** and produces the metalloprotease, **tetanospasmin**, also known as **tetanus toxin**. The organism moves to the central nervous system, where the tetanospasmin **blocks neurotransmission** by cleaving membrane proteins involved in neuroexocytosis of GABA and glycine. This results clinically in tonic contractions of voluntary muscles, often involving muscles of the jaw that result in **trismus (lockjaw) and/or risus sardonicus (sardonic smile)**. During all of this, the patient is fully conscious and the pain may be intense. If the disease interferes with the mechanics of respiration, it can be fatal.

➤ Patients who develop symptoms of tetanus should immediately be administered muscle relaxants, sedation, and pain medications, and should be considered for mechanical ventilation. The antibiotic *penicillin* can also be administered to inhibit further toxin production.

B. Parasites

Naegleria fowleri

- Free-living amoeba

CLINICAL CORRELATES—PRIMARY AMOEBIC MENINGOENCEPHALITIS

➤ This amoeba is acquired when swimming in fresh water during hot weather (occurs mostly in kids) and can cause a rapidly progressing meningoencephalitis resulting in coma and death.

C. Viruses

La Crosse (California) Encephalitis Virus

- Bunyavirus

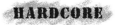

Remember that *C. tetani* is **not an invasive organism**, but rather its spores are seeded into an area of devitalized tissue, resulting in infection.

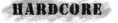

Tetanus immune globin should be administered to any patient suspected of having contact with *C. tetani* (e.g., trauma patients with open lesions or wounds) and an out-of-date vaccination status. Tetanus Ig neutralizes toxin unfixed to nervous tissue and supplies systemic protection for 2 to 4 weeks. In these patients, tetanus toxoid should be administered along with antitoxin prophylaxis at different injection sites.

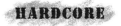

Patients with *N. fowleri* infection will have **purulent CSF with "slug-like" amoeba**.

CLINICAL CORRELATES—ENCEPHALITIS

➤ The LaCrosse virus is an encephalitis-causing arbovirus spread by mosquitos. People at risk are those who live in or visit woodland habitats, as well as those involved in outdoor recreational activities in areas where the disease is common.

IV. GASTROINTESTINAL SYSTEM

A. Parasites

Giardia lamblia

- Protozoa
- Flagellated trophozoite
- Multiple flagella

CLINICAL CORRELATES—GIARDIASIS

➤ Giardiasis is characterized by **foul-smelling and fatty diarrhea (steatorrhea)**, fever, abdominal cramps, bloating, and flatulence. G. *lamblia* is an **intestinal flagellate** that exists as both **cysts and trophozoites**. Cysts are the infectious form of the parasite, and when ingested cyst excystation occurs in the small bowel, releasing **trophozoites** (pear-shaped, binucleate, multiflagellated organisms). Trophozoites are the replicating form of the parasite. For the organism to become infectious, trophozoites must revert back to cysts within the host large intestine. **New cysts are then passed back into the environment in feces.**

➤ Waterborne transmission is mainly responsible for the transmission of giardiasis in international travelers and people hiking or camping in wilderness areas. **Surface water, such as mountain streams and municipal reservoirs, can harbor Giardia cysts** that are resistant to routine levels of chlorination. In addition, native mammals, such as **beavers**, can act as continuing sources of water contamination in natural sources of water.

  ▪ Remember: **"Beaver Fever!"**

➤ Diagnosis of G. *lamblia* requires finding cysts in formed stools, or finding both cysts and trophozoites in liquid stools by stool ELISA.

HARDCORE REVIEW TABLE—INFECTIONS OF OUTDOOR ENTHUSIASTS (TABLE 13-1)

TABLE 13-1	Infections of Outdoor Enthusiasts		
BUGS	**BUG POINTS**	**MOST COMMON PRESENTATION**	**HARDCORE MICROBIOLOGY**
Skin			
Borrelia burgdorferi	Spirochete	Lyme disease	Passed by the *Ixodes* tick found on the white-footed mouse and white-tailed deer; three stages of disease; false + VDRL (test for syphilis); visualized with Wright stain
Rickettsia rickettsii	• Gram-negative • Obligate intracellular bacterium	Rocky Mountain spotted fever	From the bite of the *Dermacentor* tick; typically presents as a rash that spreads to include the palms and soles
Sporothrix schenckii	• Dimorphic fungus • Cigar-shaped yeast	Sporotrichosis	Classically associated with a gardener who has been punctured by rose thorns; spreads along the lymphatic tract
Pulmonary System			
Blastomyces dermatitidis	• Dimorphic fungus	Blastomycosis	Pneumonia, virulence factor WI-1
Coccidioides immitis and *posadasii*	• Dimorphic yeast • Endospores	Coccidioidomycosis	Found in southwestern U.S. and northern Mexico; valley fever
Histoplasma capsulatum	• Dimorphic yeast • No capsule • Endospores	Histoplasmosis	Found in Mississippi and Ohio River basins; cultured on Sabouraud's agar; survives intracellularly

(Continued)

TABLE 13-1　Infections of Outdoor Enthusiasts (cont.)

Bugs	Bug Points	Most Common Presentation	Hardcore Microbiology
Hantavirus	• Negative-sense RNA virus • Bunyavirus • Single stranded	Hantavirus pulmonary syndrome	Carried in rodent saliva and droppings; transmitted by inhalation; >50% mortality
Nervous System			
Clostridium tetani	• Gram-positive bacteria • Possesses O (somatic) flagellar antigen • Obligate anaerobe • Spore-forming	Tetanus	Virulence factor tetanospasmin or "tetanus toxin"; clinical features include trismus (lockjaw) and risus sardonicus (sardonic smile)
Naegleria fowleri	• Free-living amoeba	Primary amebic meningoencephalitis	Acquired by swimming in fresh water; purulent CSF
La Crosse (California) encephalitis virus	• Bunyavirus	Encephalitis	Arbovirus spread by mosquitoes
Gastrointestinal System			
Giardia lamblia	• Multiple flagella • Protozoan parasite	Giardiasis	Giardia cysts found in the surface water of mountain streams and municipal reservoirs; beaver as carrier

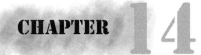
Infections Associated with Animal Contact

Zoonosis refers to any parasite-caused or infectious disease in animals that can be transmitted to humans. There are number of organisms associated with specific animal-to-human contact that frequently show up on the Step 1 examination, so be familiar with each of the following organisms and infectious diseases associated with specific animal interactions.

Bugs discussed in this chapter (Fig. 14-1):

- *Francisella tularensis*
- *Brucella*
- Western equine encephalitis virus
- Eastern equine encephalitis virus
- St. Louis encephalitis virus
- *Coxiella burnetti*
- Rabies virus
- *Bacillus anthracis*
- *Bartonella henselae*

- Toxoplasmosis
- *Echinococcus*
- West Nile virus
- *Chlamydia psittaci*
- *Ehrlichia*
- *Pasteurella multocida*
- *Yersina enterocolitica*
- *Yersinia pestis*
- *Leptospira interrogans*

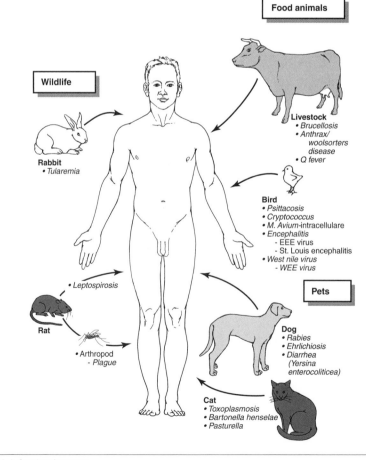

Figure 14–1 Overview of zoonoses.

I. LIVESTOCK

A. Gram-Positive Bacteria

Bacillus anthracis

- Gram-positive rod
- Aerobe
- Endospores

CLINICAL CORRELATES—ANTHRAX, WOOL-SORTER'S DISEASE

➤ *B. anthracis* is a nonmotile, sporulating gram-positive rod that causes three anthrax syndromes: *cutaneous, inhalation, and gastrointestinal anthrax*. *B. anthracis* is a natural component of the soil that initially infects grazing animals by ingestion. *Sporulating B. anthracis* can then be transferred to humans via *contaminated animal hides, or directly through the inhalation of existing spores in the soil*.

➤ *Inhalation anthrax*, or Wool-Sorter's disease, follows the inhalation of anthrax spores generated during the cleaning of contaminated goat hair.

➤ Spores of virulent *B. anthracis* can also be introduced *subcutaneously*. After entry into the skin, *B. anthracis's* **antiphagocytic capsule** facilitates local spread, while its release of an **exotoxin** results in edema, tissue necrosis, shock, and respiratory distress.

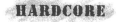

HARDCORE

Anthrax infection combines three exotoxins: edema factor, lethal factor, and protective antigen.

B. Gram-Negative Bacteria

Brucella

- Gram-negative bacillus
- Facultative intracellular parasite

CLINICAL CORRELATES—BRUCELLOSIS

➤ Brucellosis is characterized by the development of a fever, profound muscle weakness, and the formation of *granulomas* within the spleen, liver, and bone marrow.

➤ This illness is most commonly seen in *livestock farmers, veterinarians, and meat processors*.

Coxiella burnetii

- Gram negative
- Obligate intracellular parasite

CLINICAL CORRELATES—Q FEVER

➤ *Coxiella* is spread to humans by aerosols from cattle, goats, and sheep and causes Q fever. Q fever most commonly presents as a self-limited, flu-like illness, but has also been associated with interstitial pneumonia, hepatosplenomegaly, myocarditis, endocarditis, and encephalitis.

➤ *Coxiella* is an obligate intracellular organism that replicates in the cytoplasm.

II. DOGS

A. Bacteria

Ehrlichia canis

- Obligate intracellular parasite

CLINICAL CORRELATES—EHRLICHIOSIS

➤ Ehrlichiosis is a mild disease with patients complaining of malaise, headache, and rash (in 20% of patients).

➤ *Ehrlichia* are obligate intracellular bacteria that grow within membrane-bound vacuoles in human and animal leukocytes.

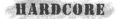

HARDCORE

Ehrlichial inclusion bodies in leukocytes are seen in blood smears containing *Ehrlichia*.

Yersinia enterocolitica

- Gram-negative rod
- Non-lactose fermenter

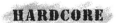

- Facultative intracellular organism
- Facultative anaerobe

CLINICAL CORRELATES—DIARRHEA

➤ *Y. enterocolitica* is transmitted via *pet feces, typically from puppies*. Most commonly, this infection occurs in outbreaks among the pediatric population. Infection can result in fever, leukocytosis and microabcess formation.

➤ *Yersinia* has a distinctive bipolar staining that gives a *safety-pin appearance* under microscopy.

B. Viruses

Rabies virus

- Negative, single-stranded RNA virus
- *Rhabdoviridiae*

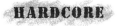

CLINICAL CORRELATES—RABIES

➤ A wide variety of animals act as a reservoir for the rabies virus, but the most commonly tested include *dogs, cats, and bats*. After human inoculation via animal bite, the rabies virus *travels along the axoplasm of peripheral neurons* toward the brain. If left untreated, the infection is fatal, resulting in encephalitis and neuronal degeneration of the brain and spinal cord.

➤ Produces specific cytoplasmic inclusion bodies in infected cells called **Negri bodies**.

III. CATS

Bartonella henselae

- Gram-negative
- Not an obligate intracellular parasite

CLINICAL CORRELATES—CAT-SCRATCH DISEASE

➤ Cat-scratch disease follows a *cat bite or scratch* and is characterized by small abscesses and cutaneous and lymph node disease at the site of injury.

Pasteurella multocida

- Gram-negative rod
- Facultative anaerobe

CLINICAL CORRELATES—PASTEURELLA

➤ *Pasteurella* lives in the upper respiratory tract and oral cavity of *felines and fowl*. Following an infected animal bite or scratch, patients develop an intense inflammatory *cellulitis* that may progress to *septic arthritis or osteomyelitis*. Meningitis, intra-abdominal infection, or endocarditis are other possible sequelae.

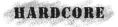

Toxoplasma gondii

- Protozoa
- Obligate intracellular parasite
- Trophozoites
- Oocyst

CLINICAL CORRELATES—TOXOPLASMOSIS

➤ *T. gondii* is a protozoa that uses cats as hosts and can be transmitted to humans from *cat feces*, resulting in neonatal infections in pregnant women and CNS mass lesions in immunocompromised patients.

IV. BIRDS

A. Bacteria

Chlamydia psittaci

- Gram-negative
- Obligate intracellular parasite

CLINICAL CORRELATES—PSITTACOSIS

➤ *C. psittaci* commonly infects birds, particularly *parrots and poultry*. This bug can be spread to humans resulting in lower respiratory tract infection and pneumonia.

➤ As an obligate intracellular pathogen, *Chlamydia* *is unable to synthesize ATP* and *divides by binary fission* in intracellular vacuoles.

B. Viruses

Eastern Equine Encephalitis Virus (EEE)

* Positive, single-stranded RNA virus
* *Togaviridae* (alpha virus)
* Icosahedral nucleocapsid
* Arbovirus

CLINICAL CORRELATES—ENCEPHALITIS

➤ In North America, wild birds and swamp mosquitoes maintain the EEE virus. Infection begins with fever, headache, nausea, and vomiting before neurological symptoms develop that lead to coma, seizures, and cranial nerve palsies.

St. Louis Encephalitis Virus (SLEV)

* Positive, single-stranded RNA virus
* *Flaviviridae*
* Nonsegmental

CLINICAL CORRELATES—ENCEPHALITIS

➤ The principal reservoirs of SLEV include *wild birds and domestic fowl*; however, the virus is transmitted to humans by *mosquitoes*. Clinical manifestations of SLEV infection range from flu-like syndromes to fatal encephalitis.

West Nile Nirus

* Positive-stranded, RNA virus
* *Flavivirdae*

CLINICAL CORRELATES—ENCEPHALITIS, MENINGOENCEPHALITIS

➤ West Nile virus (WNV) is a flavivirus that infects fibroblasts, vascular endothelial cells, and cells of the reticuloendothelial system. This virus is maintained in a bird—mosquito—bird cycle in which *birds act as the primary amplifying host*. Human infections follow the bite of infected mosquitoes, resulting in WNV viremia and subsequent central nervous system infection with *signs of encephalitis associated with muscle weakness and flaccid paralysis*.

➤ The peak incidence of WNV infection is late summer and early fall.

Western Equine Encephalitis Virus (WEE)

* Positive, single-stranded RNA virus
* *Togaviridae* (alpha virus)

CLINICAL CORRELATES—ENCEPHALITIS

➤ WEE is an arthropod-borne viral found in the Americas. This *infection occurs in areas of heightened water levels*, particularly with episodes of flooding that increase viral-carrying mosquito breeding. Although both children and adults can acquire WEE, neurological sequelae are more common in infants and may be fatal.

➤ WEE is diagnosed by isolating IgM antibody from CSF and IgG antibodies from serum.

V. RABBITS

Francisella tularensis

* Gram-negative rod
* Obligate aerobe
* Facultative intracellular parasite

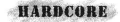

In EEE infection, cerebrospinal fluid analysis will show *pleocytosis with neutrophilic predominance* and *elevated protein concentration*, while serum testing demonstrates leukocytosis and hyponatremia.

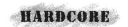

Although known as the "St. Louis" encephalitis virus, outbreaks of infection from this virus are widely distributed across the United States.

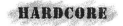

Diagnosis of WNV infection is made by isolating IgM in serum or CSF. These patients will also require a lumbar puncture, electromyography, and nerve conduction studies.

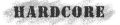

F. tularensis will grow on media of chocolate and Thayer-Martin.

CLINICAL CORRELATES—TULAREMIA

➤ Tularemia is characterized by an abrupt onset of fever, chills, shortness of breath, lymphadenopathy, and possible death that follows a tick bite from an infected animal, most notably **rabbits** or deer.

VI. RODENTS

A. Bacteria

Leptospira interrogans

- Gram-negative spirochete
- Aerobic

CLINICAL CORRELATES—LEPTOSPIROSIS

➤ *Leptospira* is transmitted to humans via water or food contaminated with animal urine or feces, most commonly from **rat urine**. Spirochetes invade the liver, kidneys, and CNS via hematogenous spread, which may develop into jaundice, hemorrhage, tissue necrosis, and possibly aseptic meningitis.

Yersinia pestis

- Gram-negative rod
- Non-lactose fermenter
- Facultative intracellular organism
- Facultative anaerobe

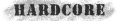

Plague-associated subcutaneous hemorrhage leads to blackish skin discoloration, which is why plague is called "black death."

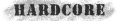

Yersinia's virulence factors are only expressed at 37°C (temperature-sensitive).

CLINICAL CORRELATES—PLAGUE

➤ *Y. pestis* is an organism that primarily affects rodents and fleas but can infect humans via bites by rodent fleas, exposure to people infected with pneumonic plague, the handling of infected animal carcasses, or exposure to aerosols, resulting in the plague.

➤ Plague is characterized by the sudden onset of fever, chills, weakness, and headache quickly followed by an intense pain in a lymph node-bearing area, most commonly the inguinal region. This is called a **bubo**, which is characterized by exquisite tenderness without fluctuation along with erythema and edema of the overlying skin. Long-term complications include vascular collapse and disseminated intravascular coagulation.

➤ Diagnosis is made by **bipolar Gram staining** in which the ends of the rod stain darker due to increased stain uptake.

HARDCORE REVIEW TABLES—INFECTIONS FROM ANIMAL CONTACT (TABLE 14-1 TO TABLE 14-6)

TABLE 14-1 Livestock			
BUGS	**BUG POINTS**	**MOST COMMON PRESENTATION**	**HARDCORE MICROBIOLOGY**
Gram-Positive Bacteria			
Bacillus anthracis	• Gram-positive rod • Aerobe • Endospores	Anthrax, Wool Sorter's disease	Three anthrax syndromes: cutaneous, inhalation, and gastrointestinal; sporulating; transferred to humans via contaminated animal hides or inhalation of existing spores in the soil; release of exotoxin results in edema, tissue necrosis, shock, and respiratory distress
Gram-Negative Bacteria			
Brucella	• Gram-negative bacillus • Facultative intracellular parasite	Brucellosis • Granulomas within the spleen, liver, and bone marrow	Seen in livestock farmers, veterinarians, and meat processors
Coxiella burnetii	• Gram-negative • Obligate intracellular parasite	Q fever • Interstitial pneumonia • Hepatosplenomegaly • Myocarditis • Endocarditis • Encephalitis	Spread to humans by aerosols from cattle, goats, and sheep

TABLE 14-2 Dogs

Bugs	Bug Points	Most Common Presentation	Hardcore Microbiology
Bacteria			
Ehrlichia canis	• Obligate intracellular parasite	Ehrlichiosis • Malaise • Headache • Rash	Obligate intracellular bacteria that grow within membrane-bound vacuoles in human and animal leukocytes; on blood smear will see ehrichial inclusion bodies in leukocytes
Yersina enterocolitica	• Gram-negative rod • Non-lactose fermenter • Facultative intracellular organism • Facultative anaerobe	Diarrhea	Transmitted via pet feces, typically from puppies; bipolar staining gives safetypin appearance under microscopy
Viruses			
Rabies virus	• Negative, single-stranded RNA virus • *Rhabdoviridiae*	Rabies • Encephalitis • Neuronal degeneration of the brain and spinal cord	Common reservoirs include dogs, cats, and bats; travels along the axoplasm of peripheral neurons toward the brain; replicates in cytoplasm

TABLE 14-3 Cats

Bugs	Bug Points	Most Common Presentation	Hardcore Microbiology
Bartonella henselae	• Gram-negative • Not obligate intracellular parasite	Cat-scratch disease • Abscesses • Cutaneous and lymph node disease at the site of injury	Follows a cat bite or scratch
Pasteurella multocida	• Gram-negative rod • Facultative anaerobe	Pasteurella • Inflammatory cellulitis • Possible septic arthritis or osteomyelitis	Found in felines and fowl
Toxoplasma gondii	• Protozoa • Obligate intracellular parasite • Trophozoites • Oocyst	Toxoplasmosis • Neonatal infections • CNS mass lesions (immunocompromised)	Transmitted to humans via cat feces

TABLE 14-4 Birds

Bugs	Bug Points	Most Common Presentation	Hardcore Microbiology
Gram-Negative Bacteria			
Chlamydia psittaci	• Gram-negative • Obligate intracellular parasite	Psittacosis • Lower respiratory tract infection • Pneumonia	Natural infectious organism of birds, particularly parrots and poultry; unable to synthesize ATP; divides by binary fission
Viruses			
Eastern equine encephalitis virus	• Positive, single-stranded RNA virus • *Togaviridae* (alpha virus) • Icosahedral nucleocapsid • Arbovirus	Encephalitis	Wild birds and swamp mosquitoes maintain the EEE virus; cerebrospinal fluid analysis will show pleocytosis with neutrophilic predominance and elevated protein concentration; replicates in cytoplasm
St. Louis encephalitis virus	• Positive, single-stranded RNA virus • *Flaviviridae* • Nonsegmental	Encephalitis	Transmitted to humans by mosquitoes; principal reservoirs are wild birds and domestic fowl
West Nile virus	• Positive-stranded, RNA virus • *Flavivirdae*	Encephalitis, meningoencephalitis	Infects fibroblasts, vascular endothelial cells, and cells of the reticuloendothelial system; birds act as the primary amplifying host; diagnosis by isolating IgM antibodies
Western equine encephalitis virus	• Positive, single-stranded RNA virus • *Togaviridae* (alpha virus)	Encephalitis	Occurs in areas of heightened water levels that increase viral-carrying mosquito breeding

TABLE 14-5 Rabbits

Bugs	Bug Points	Most Common Presentation	Hardcore Microbiology
Francisella tularensis	• Gram-negative rod • Obligate aerobe • Facultative intracellular parasite	Tularemia • Fever • Chills • Headache • Malaise	Classically follows exposure to an infected rabbit; grows on chocolate and Thayer-Martin media

TABLE 14-6 Rodents

Bugs	Bug Points	Most Common Presentation	Hardcore Microbiology
Leptospira interrogans	• Gram-negative spirochete • Aerobic	Leptospirosis • Jaundice • Hemorrhage • Tissue necrosis • Aseptic meningitis	Transmitted to humans via water or food contaminated with rat urine; invades the liver, kidneys, and CNS
Yersinia pestis	• Gram-negative rod • Non-lactose fermenter • Facultative intracellular organism • Facultative anaerobe	Plague • Vascular collapse • Disseminated intravascular coagulation • Bubo development	Infects humans via bites by rodent fleas; commonly associated with bubos; bipolar Gram staining for diagnosis; temperature-sensitive virulence factors

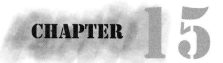

Infections of the Underdeveloped World

People living in underdeveloped areas of the world are prone to infections caused by poor sanitation, poor hygiene, and limited access to vaccinations and pharmaceuticals. Be on the lookout for the following bugs if a question stem includes any underdeveloped regions, foreign travelers, or mention of new immigrants.

Bugs discussed in this chapter:

- Epstein-Barr virus
- Polio
- *Mycobacterium leprae*
- *Leishmania*
- Ebola virus
- Marburg virus
- *Borrelia recurrentis*
- *Treponema pallidum*

- *Shigella dysenteriae*
- *Campylobacter jejuni*
- *Mycobacterium tuberculosis*
  Vibrio cholerae
- *Chlamydia trachomatis*
- *Rickettsia prowazekii* and *Rickettsia typhi*
- *Trypanosoma brucei*
- *Trypanosoma cruzi*

I. BACTERIA

Borrelia recurrentis

- Gram-negative spirochete
- Microaerophilic

CLINICAL CORRELATES—RELAPSING FEVER

> Relapsing fever, caused by the *Borrelia* genus, is an arthropod-borne infection which occurs in two major forms: **tick-borne (TBRF) and louse-borne (LBRF)**. Louse-borne relapsing fever is typically seen in the developing world and is transmitted from person to person via louse infestations secondary to poor hygiene, overcrowded conditions, and poor sanitation.

> Relapsing fever is characterized by recurrent episodes of fever that present with the sudden onset of fever followed by several afebrile periods. Other symptoms include neck stiffness, myalgias, and nausea that may accompany episodes of fever.

Campylobacter jejuni

- Gram-negative rod
- Oxidase-positive

CLINICAL CORRELATES—CAMPYLOBACTER ENTERITIS

> *Campylobacter* is the leading cause of acute diarrhea worldwide, and is transmitted primarily by eating poultry, drinking surface water, or drinking unpasteurized milk. *Campylobacter* infection causes **bloody diarrhea**.

> Remember that *Campylobacter* has an enterotoxin that acts in a similar manner to cholera toxin, as well as a cytotoxin that acts on mucosal cells.

Chlamydia trachomatis

- Gram-negative
- Obligate intracellular parasite

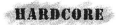

HARDCORE

Other than *Borrelia recurrentis* (transmitted by the louse), relapsing fever caused by *Borrelia* spp. is transmitted by ticks.

HARDCORE

Borrelia is able to vary its expression of outer membrane lipoproteins (**antigenic variation**), which enables the organism to escape from immune-mediated opsonization and phagocytosis.

CLINICAL CORRELATES—TRACHOMA: CONJUNCTIVITIS AND BLINDNESS

➢ *C. trachomatis* causes trachoma, a form of conjunctivitis which, is *the leading cause of preventable blindness in the world*. This infection occurs in children in underdeveloped areas of the world. Transmission of *C. trachomatis* occurs during newborn delivery through an infected birth canal or by hand-to-hand transfer of infected eye secretions. Infection results in *inflammation and scar formation of the eyelid*, causing the eyelashes to fold inward towards the eye. Ultimately, the inwardly displaced eyelashes rub against the cornea, leading to blindness if left untreated.

➢ Diagnosis requires the demonstration of *intracytoplasmic basophilic inclusion bodies* in cells taken from the palpebral conjunctival surface.

Rickettsia prowazekii and *Rickettsia typhi*

- Gram-negative
- Obligate intracellular bacterium

CLINICAL CORRELATES—EPIDEMIC TYPHUS (CAUSED BY RICKETTSIA PROWAZEKII) AND MURINE TYPHUS (CAUSED BY RICKETTSIA TYPHI)

➢ Typhus is a potentially lethal infection characterized by the abrupt onset of fever, headache, and rash followed by the development of CNS sequelae that may include confusion, drowsiness, coma, or seizures.

➢ Both forms of typhus are present in sub-Saharan Africa. *Epidemic typhus (Rickettsia prowazekii) is transmitted by the body louse*. This infection typically occurs in conditions that favor the proliferation of lice, such as during war or natural disasters.

➢ *Murine typhus is transmitted to humans by rat or cat fleas* and occurs most commonly in urban settings.

Shigella dysenteriae

- Gram-negative rod
- Beta-hemolytic
- Non-lactose fermenter
- Indole +

CLINICAL CORRELATES—BACTERIAL DIARRHEA

➢ *S. dysenteriae* is rare in the United States and is typically found in developing countries. *Shigella* invades colonic enterocytes and causes *bloody, mucoid darrhea*. *Shigella* is spread directly from person to person and from contaminated food and water.

➢ The *Shigella* toxin, called *shiga toxin*, inhibits protein synthesis and kills intestinal cells.

➢ Remember that the *Shigella* organism is *nonmotile*, while the *Salmonella* organism is *highly motile*.

Treponema pertenue

- Gram-negative, corkscrew shaped
- Spirochete

CLINICAL CORRELATES—YAWS

➢ Yaws is a contagious, nonvenereal infection that typically occurs in children younger than 15 years old in tropical areas of Africa, Asia, and South America.

➢ *T. pertenue* infection presents as an ulcerative skin lesion that contains a large concentration of spirochetes. Similar to syphilis, yaws can be classified into three stages as the disease disseminates from cutaneous lesions to cause bone, joint, and soft tissue deformities.

➢ *T. pertenue* may be transmitted via direct skin-to-skin contact and through breaks in the skin from trauma, bites, or excoriations.

Vibrio cholerae

- Gram-negative rod
- Oxidase +
- Ferments sugars except lactose

CLINICAL CORRELATES—CHOLERA

➤ Cholera is characterized by severe, *watery diarrhea*, which rapidly produces dehydration and leads to death in more than 50% of untreated patients.

➤ *V. cholera* contains a cholera toxin that binds to the surface of enterocytes and leads to an *elevation in cyclic AMP* within the intestinal mucosa (same toxin as the LT toxin in ETEC). This elevated cAMP causes an increase in chloride secretion, a reduction in sodium absorption, and massive loss of fluid and electrolytes via severe watery diarrhea and vomiting. As stools become watery with flecks of mucus, they may be described as *"rice water" stools*.

➤ Cholera occurs in the developing countries of Asia and Africa, and regions of South and Central America.

II. MYCOBACTERIUM

Mycobacterium leprae

- Acid-fast rod
- Catalase +
- Phenolase +
- Facultative intracellular growth
- Aerobic

CLINICAL CORRELATES—LEPROSY

➤ M. *leprae* infection primarily affects superficial tissues, specifically the skin and peripheral nerves. Two forms of the disease exist:

1. *Tuberculoid form*—Involves the skin and peripheral nerves. These patients have *a vigorous cellular immune response* to the organism.

2. *Lepromatous form*—Characterized by extensive skin involvement. These patients have a *minimal cellular immune response*.

Mycobacterium tuberculosis

- Acid-fast rod
- Catalase +
- Aerobic

CLINICAL CORRELATES—TUBERCULOSIS

➤ Parts of the world with the highest incidence of tuberculosis include sub-Saharan Africa, India, China, and Southeast Asia.

III. PARASITES

Leishmania donovani and Leishmania chagasi

- Protozoan

CLINICAL CORRELATES—LEISHMANIASIS

➤ Leishmaniasis is spread by the bite of a *female sandfly*, in which the parasite is injected into the skin and taken up by macrophages. Infected macrophages can remain in the skin and cause cutaneous disease, or they can disseminate, producing visceral disease consisting of organomegaly, fever, cachexia, pancytopenia, and hypergammaglobulinemia.

Trypanosoma rhodesiense and Trypanosoma gambiense (African)

- Protozoan

CLINICAL CORRELATES—SLEEPING SICKNESS (HUMAN AFRICAN TRYPANOSOMIASIS)

➤ *Trypanosoma brucei* parasites are transmitted to humans by the *tsetse fly*.

➤ Symptoms of infection begin with the development of an inflammatory lesion called a **trypanosomal chancre** at the site of the bite along with a fever, headache, and rash. If untreated,

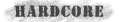

V. cholera is **comma shaped**, with a single polar flagellum.

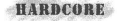

Leprosy is found in wild armadillos in the south-central United States.

HARDCORE

The diagnosis of leprosy is made by identifying *M. leprae*'s ability to convert dopa into pigmentation products (phenolase +).

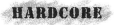

There are two regional forms of sleeping sickness. Along with the Eastern Africa-associated *T. rhodesiense*, sleeping sickness in the Western and Central Africa is caused by *Trypanosoma gambiense*.

infection can progress to meningoencephalitis, cerebral hemorrhages, and widespread multifocal white matter demyelination. At this later stage, patients develop difficulty concentrating, personality changes, and psychosis, worsening until *coma and death ultimately occur*.

Trypanosoma cruzi (American)

- Protozoan

CLINICAL CORRELATES—CHAGAS' DISEASE (AMERICAN TRYPANOSOMIASIS)

➤ Chagas' disease is found only in Central and South America, Mexico, and the southern United States, and is associated with serious complications including *dilated cardiomyopathy, megaesophagus, and megacolon*. Cardiac involvement is characterized by myocarditis, as well as *dilated cardiomyopathy*.

➤ The life-cycle of *T. cruzi* consists of three stages and involves mammalian reservoirs including rodents, opossums, armadillos, and raccoons, but is passed to humans by the *reduviid bug*. When this bug takes a blood meal from a human host, it defecates around the bite site. The resulting irritation causes the host to scratch the site and contaminate the wound with parasites discharged in the feces.

IV. VIRUSES

Ebola Virus

- Negative, single-stranded RNA virus
- *Filoviridae*
- Nonsegmented

CLINICAL CORRELATES—EBOLA HEMORRHAGIC FEVER

➤ Ebola hemorrhagic fever occurs in sub-Saharan Africa and infection includes a mortality rate of up to 90%. Transmission occurs through direct contact with body fluid from infected individuals. Currently, the natural reservoir of Ebola virus is unknown.

Epstein-Barr Virus (EBV)

- Double-stranded, linear DNA virus
- Herpesvirus
- Icosahedral nucleocapsid

CLINICAL CORRELATES—BURKITT'S LYMPHOMA

➤ Burkitt's lymphoma is characterized by a *tumor that localizes to the jaw*. It is the most common *childhood malignancy in Africa*.

Marburg Virus

- Negative, single-stranded RNA virus
- *Filoviridae*
- Nonsegmented

CLINICAL CORRELATES—MARBURG HEMORRHAGIC FEVER

➤ Transmission of the Marburg virus occurs with contact of infected bodily secretion, including close contact with dead people. Marburg hemorrhagic fever has a *high mortality rate and causes death by multi-organ failure*.

Poliovirus

- Positive, single-stranded RNA virus
- *Enteroviridae*

CLINICAL CORRELATES—POLIO

➤ Polio is a RNA virus that infects human anterior horn cells of the spinal cord, causing a variety of illnesses that range from an asymptomatic infection to *aseptic meningitis and paralytic poliomyelitis*. The virus is spread *fecal–orally* (and less so via respiratory secretions), and initially replicates in the *tonsils and Peyer's patches of the small intestine*. Once the infection migrates to the spinal cord, it targets anterior horn cells and destroys presynaptic motor neurons and postsynaptic neurons that exit at that location. Paralytic poliomyelitis is characterized by *peripheral motor neuron defects* caused by damage to exiting motor neurons, and *central motor neuron defects* with damage to the presynaptic neurons.

➤ Two vaccinations are used worldwide:

- **Inactivated polio vaccine (Salk)**—Formalin-killed viruses are injected subcutaneously, initiating an IgG antibody response.
- **Oral polio vaccine (Sabin)**—An attenuated poliovirus that cannot multiply in the CNS is ingested orally. This form of vaccination induces the formation of IgG in the blood and IgA in the intestines, but also has the potential to pick up virulence and cause clinical sequelae (very rare).

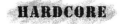

HARDCORE

More than 90% of patients exposed to poliovirus are asymptomatic. Less than 2% of all people exposed to the virus develop paralytic symptoms.

HARDCORE REVIEW TABLES—INFECTIONS OF THE UNDERDEVELOPED WORLD (TABLE 15-1 TO TABLE 15-4)

TABLE 15-1 Bacteria

BUGS	BUG POINTS	MOST COMMON PRESENTATION	HARDCORE MICROBIOLOGY
Borrelia recurrentis	• Gram-negative spirochete • Microaerophilic	Relapsing fever • Recurrent episodes of fever • Neck stiffness • Myalgias • Nausea	Antigenic variation, louse-borne, transmitted via louse infestation secondary to poor hygiene, overcrowded conditions, and poor sanitation
Campylobacter jejuni	• Gram-negative rod • Oxidase positive	*Campylobacter* enteritis • Bloody diarrhea	Leading cause of acute diarrhea worldwide; transmitted by poultry, drinking surface water, or raw milk
Chlamydia trachomatis	• Gram-negative • Obligate intracellular parasite	Trachoma: • Conjunctivitis • Blindness	Leading cause of preventable blindness in the world; diagnosis requires intracytoplasmic basophilic inclusion bodies in cells from palpebral conjunctival surface
Rickettsia prowazekii and *Rickettsia typhi*	• Gram-negative • Obligate intracellular bacterium	Epidemic typhus (*Rickettsia prowazekii*) and murine typhus (*Rickettsia typhi*) • Fever • Rash • CNS sequelae (confusion, coma, seizures)	Epidemic typhus is transmitted by the body louse; murine typhus is transmitted by rat or cat fleas
Shigella dysenteriae	• Gram-negative rod • Beta-hemolytic • Non-lactose fermenter • Indole +	Bacterial diarrhea • Bloody, mucoid diarrhea	Spread by direct person-to-person contact, as well as from contaminated food and water
Treponema pertenue	• Gram-negative, corkscrew shaped • Spirochete	Yaws • Ulcerative skin lesion	Occurs in children under 15 years of age in tropical areas of Africa, Asia, and South America
Vibrio cholerae	• Gram-negative rod • Oxidase + • Ferments sugars except lactose	Cholera • Watery diarrhea	Cholera toxin binds to enterocytes, elevates cAMP within intestinal mucosa, increasing chloride secretion and reducing sodium absorption, "rice water" stools

TABLE 15-2 Mycobacterium

BUGS	BUG POINTS	MOST COMMON PRESENTATION	HARDCORE MICROBIOLOGY
Mycobacterium leprae	• Acid-fast rod • Catalase + • Phenolase + • Facultative intracellular growth • Aerobic	Leprosy	Affects superficial tissues (e.g., skin and peripheral nerves); found in wild armadillos in the south-central U.S.
Mycobacterium tuberculosis	• Acid-fast rod • Catalase + • Aerobic	Tuberculosis	Reactivation of primary disease occurs in lung apices; caseating necrosis; Ghon complex and nodular granulomas

TABLE 15-3 Parasites

BUGS	BUG POINTS	MOST COMMON PRESENTATION	HARDCORE MICROBIOLOGY
Leishmania donovani, L. chagasi	• Protozoan	Leishmaniasis • Organomegaly • Fever • Cachexia • Pancytopenia • Hypergammaglobulinemia	Spread by the bite of a female sandfly; infects macrophages
Trypanosoma rhodesiense and *gambiense* (African)	• Protozoan	Sleeping sickness (Human African trypanosomiasis) • Inflammatory lesion • Fever • Rash Can progress to: • Cerebral hemorrhages • Meningoencephalitis • Coma • Death	Transmitted to humans by the tsetse fly, inflammatory lesion at bite site called "try-panosomal chancre"
Trypanosoma cruzi (American)	Protozoan	Chagas' disease (American trypanosomiasis) • Cardiac disease • Megaesophagus • Megacolon	Passed to humans by the reduviid bug; cardiac involvement includes myocarditis and dilated cardiomyopathy

TABLE 15-4 Viruses

BUGS	BUG POINTS	MOST COMMON PRESENTATION	HARDCORE MICROBIOLOGY
Ebola virus	• Negative, single-stranded RNA virus • Filoviridae • Nonsegmented	Ebola hemorrhagic fever • Diffuse hemorrage from all orifices • Severe fever	Mortality rate 90%; transmission through direct contact with body fluid, replicates in cytoplasm
Epstein-Barr virus	• Double-stranded, linear DNA virus • Herpesvirus • Icosahedral nucleocapsid	Burkitt's lymphoma	Localizes to the jaw; most common childhood malignancy in Africa
Marburg virus	• Negative, single-stranded RNA virus • *Filoviridae* • Nonsegmented	Marburg hemorrhagic fever • Diffuse hemorrage from all orifices • Severe fever	High mortality rate; transmission through direct contact with body fluid; replicates in cytoplasm
Poliovirus	• Positive, single-stranded RNA virus • *Enteroviridae*	Polio • Aseptic meningitis • Paralytic poliomyelitis (motor)	Replicates in cytoplasm, spread fecal–orally, targets anterior horn cells and destroys presynaptic motor neurons and exiting postsynaptic neurons; two vaccinations are • **Inactivated polio vaccine (Salk)**—formalin-killed viruses are injected subcutaneously • **Oral polio vaccine (Sabin)**—an attenuated poliovirus ingested orally

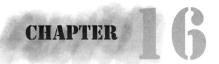

CHAPTER 16

Infections Caused by Worms (Helminths)

Helminths are parasitic worms that cause disease in humans. Two main major groups of helminths are responsible for human infection: (1) the Nematoda, or roundworms; and (2) Platyhelminthes, or flatworms, which are further categorized into trematodes (flukes) and cestodes (a.k.a. tapeworms). Because most of these infections occur outside of the United States, these bugs are not heavily emphasized on Step 1. However, you should be aware of the key differences between each species, including vectors, mechanism of infection, and clinical manifestations.

Bugs discussed in this chapter:

- *Ascaris lumbricoides*
- *Enterobius vermicularis*
- *Toxocara canis*
- *Trichuris trichiura*
- *Trichinella spiralis*
- *Ancylostoma braziliense*
- *Ancylostoma duodenale*
- *Necator americanus*
- *Strongyloides stercoralis*
- *Onchocerca volvulus*
- *Wuchereria bancrofti*

- *Loa loa*
- *Dracunculus medinensis*
- *Clonorchis sinensis*
- *Schistosoma japonicum, S. mansoni, S. haematobium*
- *Paragonimus westermani*
- *Diphyllobothrium latum*
- *Echinococcus granulosus*
- *Taenia solium*
- *Taenia saginata*

I. NEMATODES (ROUNDWORMS)

Nematodes are roundworms that are divided into:

1. *Intestinal nematodes*—Mature from eggs or larvae into adult worms within the human intestinal tract (Fig. 16-1).
   ○ *Ascaris lumbricoides, Enterobius vermicularis, Necator americanus, Strongyloides stercoralis, Trichinella spiralis, Trichuris trichiura*
2. *Blood and tissue nematodes*—Live in human blood, lymphatic fluid, and tissue (Fig. 16-2).
   ○ *Ancylostoma braziliense, Ancylostoma duodenale, Dracunculus medinensis, Onchocerca volvulus, Toxocara canis, Wuchereria bancrofti*

A key distinguishing feature of these worms is their *route of entry* into the human host:

- *Egg ingestion*—*Ascaris lumbricoides, Enterobius vermicularis, Toxocara canis, Trichuris trichiura*
- *Larvae ingestion*—*Dracunculus medinensis, Trichinella spiralis*
- *Larvae skin penetration*—*Ancylostoma braziliense, Ancylostoma duodenale, Necator americanus, Strongyloides stercoralis*
- *Arthropod vector*—*Loa loa, Onchocerca volvulus, Wuchereria bancrofti*

A. Nematodes Acquired via Egg Ingestion

Ascaris lumbricoides

CLINICAL CORRELATES—INTESTINAL INFECTION

➤ *A. lumbricoides* causes an intestinal infection, which is transmitted by the ingestion of its eggs (fecal–oral).

➤ Diagnosis is made by examination for eggs visible in the feces of infected patients.

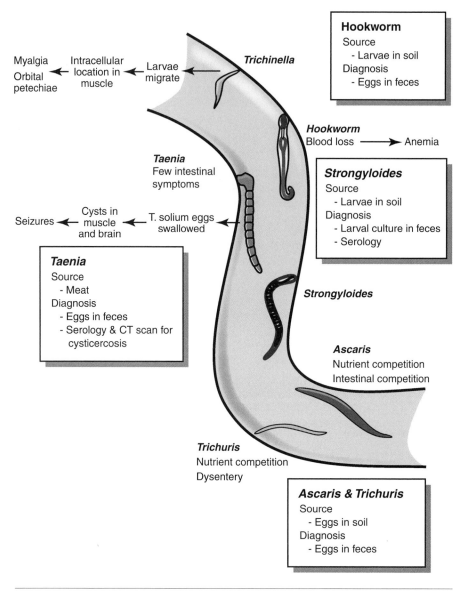

Figure 16–1 Gut helminths.

Enterobius vermicularis

CLINICAL CORRELATES—PINWORM INFECTION (INTESTINAL)

➤ Pinworm infections mainly occur in children and are characterized by intense **nighttime peri-anal itching** (pruritus ani). Transmission occurs by the ingestion of eggs (fecal–oral) and diagnosis is made by the **"Scotch tape" test**.

Toxocara canis

CLINICAL CORRELATES—VISCERAL LARVA MIGRANS/TOXOCARIASIS (BLOOD AND TISSUE NEMATODE).

➤ T. canis infection follows the ingestion of dog roundworm larvae. This worm migrates through the human body causing fever, diarrhea, and possibly hepatitis. Larvae of dog roundworm do not mature in humans.

Trichuris trichiuria

CLINICAL CORRELATES—WHIPWORM INFECTION (INTESTINAL)

➤ Whipworm infection is an intestinal infection characterized by acute abdominal pain and diarrhea after the ingestion of T. trichiuria eggs (Fig. 16-3).

➤ Diagnosis: fecal exam for eggs.

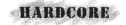

Pinworm infection from *E. vermicularis* does not cause eosinophilia.

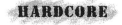

Whipworm infection *(T. trichiuria)* does not cause eosinophilia.

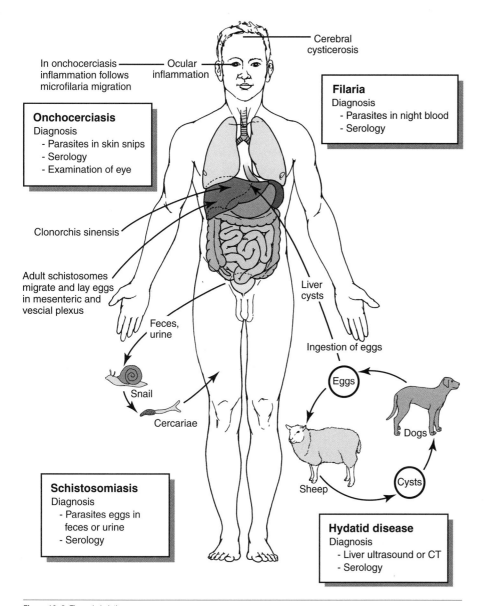

Cerebral cysticerosis

In onchocerciasis inflammation follows microfilaria migration — Ocular inflammation

Filaria
Diagnosis
 - Parasites in night blood
 - Serology

Onchocerciasis
Diagnosis
 - Parasites in skin snips
 - Serology
 - Examination of eye

Clonorchis sinensis

Adult schistosomes migrate and lay eggs in mesenteric and vescial plexus

Liver cysts

Feces, urine

Ingestion of eggs

Snail

Eggs

Dogs

Cercariae

Sheep

Cysts

Schistosomiasis
Diagnosis
 - Parasites eggs in feces or urine
 - Serology

Hydatid disease
Diagnosis
 - Liver ultrasound or CT
 - Serology

Figure 16–2 Tissue helminths.

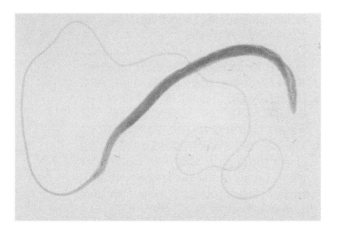

Figure 16–3 An adult worm of *T. trichiura* showing the whip configuration. The narrow portion is its anterior end. *(Reprinted with permission from Sun, Tsieh. Parasitic Disorders: Pathology, Diagnosis, and Management, 2nd edition. Baltimore: Lippincott Williams & Wilkins, 1999).*

B. Nematodes Acquired via Larvae Ingestion

Dracunculus medinensis

CLINICAL CORRELATES—BLOOD AND TISSUE NEMATODE INFECTION

> *D. medinensis* is transmitted to humans when freshwater copepods are ingested in drinking water. These larvae penetrate the intestinal lining, eventually maturing beneath the skin. When the human host immerses the area of the skin housing the worm in fresh water (e.g., while bathing in a stream), the female *D. medinensis* exposes her uterus to the environment and releases large numbers of microfilariae.

> Symptoms occur when the microfilariae are released because they are allergic in nature resulting in nausea, vomiting, and hives.

Trichinella spiralis

CLINICAL CORRELATES—INTESTINAL INFECTION

> Infection of *T. spiralis* follows the ingestion of encysted larvae typically found in *raw pork*. After larvae mature in the human or pig intestine, adult males are passed in feces while adult *females penetrate the intestinal mucosa*. While extraintestinal, females produce vast amounts of larvae that *spread to various organs and skeletal muscle via the bloodstream*, where they then become encysted.

> Clinical manifestations of infection include diarrhea, abdominal pain, and fever that are most pronounced as female worms penetrate the intestinal mucosa.

> Diagnosis by muscle biopsy and serology testing for increased levels of muscle enzymes.

C. Nematodes Acquired via Larvae Skin Penetration

Ancylostoma braziliense

CLINICAL CORRELATES—CUTANEOUS LARVA MIGRANS (BLOOD AND TISSUE NEMATODE)

> Larvae of this dog hookworm can infect humans, but mature forms of the worm cannot. Larvae penetrate the skin and cause a raised, itchy rash that advances in the epidermis along with the larvae, which is called a "*creeping eruption*."

Ancylostoma duodenale

CLINICAL CORRELATES—HOOKWORM (BLOOD AND TISSUE NEMATODE)

> Larvae of *A. duodenale* penetrate the uncovered *soles of the feet*. This infection may result in *clinical anemia*.

Necator americanus

CLINICAL CORRELATES—HOOKWORM (INTESTINAL NEMATODE)

> *N. americanus* filiform larvae penetrate the skin and travel to the alveoli of the lungs, where they are eventually coughed up and swallowed. In the intestine, hookworms reproduce and release fertilized eggs in the feces.

> Diagnosis by fecal exam for eggs.

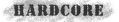

HARDCORE

D. medinensis worms are found in Africa, India, and the Middle East.

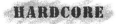

HARDCORE

Treatment of *Dracunculus* infection involves removing the worm from the skin by wrapping the parasite around a stick and pulling the creature out slowly enough not to tear the body in half (may take days). These worms can reach 100 cm in length (Fig. 16-4).

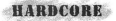

HARDCORE

Patients suffering from *Trichinella* infection will have markedly elevated eosinophil count, as well as an increase in serum muscle enzymes and creatine phospokinase as the parasites invade skeletal muscle.

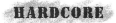

HARDCORE

N. americanus infection may result in iron-deficient anemia, as well as hemoptysis.

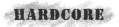

HARDCORE

Because its eggs hatch rapidly, any examination of feces for *N. americanus* eggs must take place immediately after defecation.

HARDCORE

Diagnosis of *Strongyloides* infection is by fecal exam for *larvae* (not eggs), and via the *enterotest*, in which a long nylon string is swallowed and then pulled out, showing larvae in infected patients.

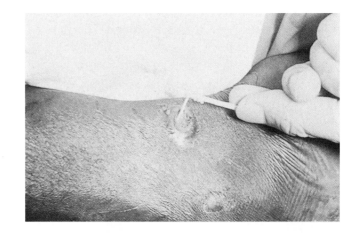

Figure 16–4 An adult female worm of *D. medinensis* is being removed by being wound onto a stick. *(Reprinted with permission from Sun, Tsieh. Parasitic Disorders: Pathology, Diagnosis, and Management, 2nd edition. Baltimore: Lippincott Williams & Wilkins, 1999).*

Strongyloides stercoralis

CLINICAL CORRELATES—INTESTINAL INFECTION

➤ *S. stercoralis* infection results after larvae penetrate skin on the feet. Like *N. americanus*, these worms *migrate to the lungs*, and then are coughed up and swallowed. After maturing in the intestine, the worm lays eggs. Some eggs are not passed in the feces, but rather the filiform larvae penetrate the intestine directly and migrate to the lung to continue the cycle. This is termed **autoinfection**. Other eggs pass in the feces to transmit infection to another host.

D. Nematodes Acquired by Arthropods

Loa loa

CLINICAL CORRELATES—LOIASIS

➤ Loiasis is caused by the filarial nematode *Loa loa*, which is transmitted to humans by day-biting *Chrysops flies*. Clinical symptoms appear when adult worms migrate to the surface of the skin, causing an immune reaction that results in diffuse *"Calabar swelling"* and granulomatous abscess formation of the arms and legs. The worms are classically known for *appearing around the eye*, and if they are not removed can cause damage to the conjunctiva (Fig. 16-5).

➤ Human loiasis occurs in the rain forest and swamp areas of West Africa.

- Remember: Loa *loa* Likes Optic Areas, and is transmitted by flies.

Onchocerca volvulus

CLINICAL CORRELATES—RIVER BLINDNESS OR ONCHOCERCIASIS (BLOOD AND TISSUE NEMATODE)

➤ *O. volvulus* is a roundworm whose offspring, or microfilariae, are spread via the *black fly*. Black flies breed in rivers and streams of Africa, Central America, and South America. After an infected fly bites a human, skin nodules develop along with a developing rash of darkened pigmentation and dry scaly skin ("lizard skin") secondary to an allergic response of the host to microfilariae. If microfilariae migrate to the eye, a strong host allergic response can lead to *blindness*.

➤ Diagnosis is via skin biopsy revealing microfilariae.

Wuchereria bancrofti

CLINICAL CORRELATES—ELEPHANTIASIS, TROPICAL PULMONARY EOSINOPHILIA (BLOOD AND TISSUE NEMATODE)

➤ *W. bancrofti* is spread via mosquito bite. Two important consequences may follow infection:

1. **Elephantiasis**—If, after repeated infections, dead filariae accumulate in lymph nodes, the lymphatic system may back up, resulting in *immense swelling and disfigurement* (including a

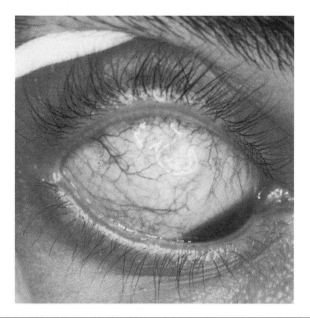

Figure 16–5 Loiasis. A threadlike *L. loa* migrating in subconjunctival tissues. *(Reprinted with permission from Gold DH and Weingeist TA. Color Atlas of the Eye in Systemic Disease. Baltimore: Lippincott Williams & Wilkins, 2001).*

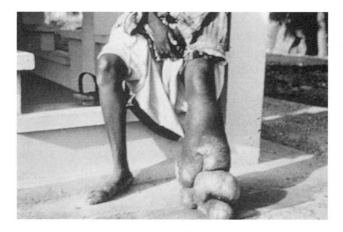

Figure 16–6 The characteristic feature of elephantiasis in the lower portion of the left leg is seen in a patient with bancroftian filariasis. *(Courtesy of Dr. H. Zaiman, Charlottesville, VA, from a pictoral presentation of parasites. From Sun, Tsieh MD. Parasitic Disorders: Pathology, Diagnosis, and Management, 2nd edition. Baltimore: Lippincott Williams & Wilkins, 1999).*

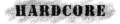

Diagnosis of *Wuchereria* infection includes the serologic examination for microfilaria in blood, which must be done at night.

substantial increase in mass of the tissue and the development of thick, scaly skin) of the lower extremities and genital areas (Fig. 16-6).

2. **Tropical pulmonary eosinophilia**—The host may develop a *hypersensitivity reaction* to filariae, resulting in bronchial constriction and hypereosinophilia.

II. PLATYHELMINTHES (FLATWORMS)

Platyhelminthes are flatworms that infect humans and can be divided into two groups:

1. **Trematodes (flukes)**—mate within humans outside of the digestive tract.
2. **Cestodes (tapeworms)**—mate within human digestive tract.

A. Trematodes (Flukes)

Clonorchis sinensis

CLINICAL CORRELATES—CHINESE LIVER FLUKE

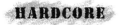

Adult Chinese liver flukes can remain in bile ducts for up to 30 years.

➤ *C. sinensis* is endemic in the Far East. This parasite is transmitted to humans in *undercooked fish* and causes *inflammation of the biliary tract* that may lead to *obstructive jaundice* resembling suppurative cholangitis.

Paragonimus westermani

CLINICAL CORRELATES—LUNG FLUKE

➤ *P. westermani* is a lung fluke that can cause pulmonary inflammation following the ingestion of undercooked crustaceans (crab).

Schistosoma japonicum, mansoni, haematobium

CLINICAL CORRELATES—SCHISTOSOMIASIS/KATAYAMA FEVER (BLOOD FLUKE)

➤ Schistosomes are trematodes that use the *freshwater snail* for multiplication. After their eggs hatch in freshwater, *Schistosoma* larvae infect and mature within the freshwater snail and then are released as *cercariae* (mature larvae) that infect humans. These parasites penetrate human skin and migrate to the *hepatic portion of the portal venous system*, where they mate. After mating, *Schistosoma eggs are laid in the bladder* of the infected human, where they can be spread to freshwater (by urinating or defecating in water) to continue the cycle. Schistosoma worms can release eggs into the venous system of human hosts, leading to portal hypertension, pulmonary hypertension, or inflammatory intestinal polyps depending on where these eggs migrate.

➤ Adult worms are not challenged by the human immune system and may exist and reproduce for years. Cercariae do activate the immune system, leading to fever, hives, cough, and weight loss.

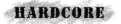

S. mansoni eggs are shaped like an oval with a spike on one end. Think of a knife, like *Charles **Manson***.

➤ Diagnosis: finding eggs in urine or stool, or ultrasound of the liver.

B. Cestodes

Diphyllobothrium latum

CLINICAL CORRELATES—FISH TAPEWORM

➤ *D. latum* is a parasite obtained from eating *larvae in freshwater fish*. Clinical manifestations include abdominal complications and *anemia caused by parasite-induced vitamin B$_{12}$ deficiency*.

➤ Diagnosis is by fecal examination for eggs and gravid proglottids.

Echinococcus granulosus

CLINICAL CORRELATES—HYDATID DISEASE

➤ *E. granulosus* eggs are found in dog feces, and human ingestion may result in *cyst formation in the lungs and liver*. After calcification, these cysts may rupture, causing cough and chest pain; or enlarge, resulting in *palpable liver masses and biliary obstruction*.

➤ Diagnosis is with CT scan or ultrasound of the liver and lung.

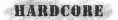

E. granulosus hydatid cysts may leak fluid, resulting in a life-threatening allergic reaction (anaphylaxis).

Taenia solium

CLINICAL CORRELATES—CYSTICERCOSIS (PORK TAPEWORM), NEUROCYSTICERCOSIS

➤ Cysticercosis is a disease acquired by the *ingestion of undercooked pork containing larvae of the tapeworm, T. solium*. This cestode contains hooks on its scolex that attach to the intestinal lining. Once attached, it releases eggs within the human GI tract that are passed with feces and then are ingested by pigs (fecal–oral). Once ingested by pigs, larvae hatch and migrate from pork intestine to muscle. After imbedding themselves in pork muscle, these larvae may be ingested by humans if pork is improperly cooked.

➤ If humans ingest *T. solium* eggs (fecal–orally) rather than larvae, these eggs hatch within the human small intestine and larvae disseminate, *traveling to muscle, the eyes, and the central nervous system*. These larvae eventually form *inflammatory, calcified cysts* within these target tissues that can lead to *blindness, seizures, and other neurological deficits (neurocysticercosis)*.

➤ This infection is diagnosed with fecal exam for eggs and gravid proglottids, as well as imaging of muscle or brain via CT scan and biopsy looking for calcified cysticerci.

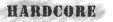

In Central and South America, as well as in Southeast Asia, cysticercosis is the most common cause of new-onset seizures.

Taenia saginata

CLINICAL CORRELATES—BEEF TAPEWORM

➤ Similar to *T. solium*, *T. saginata* are also transmitted to humans via undercooked meat; however, these cestodes are passed by the *ingestion of larvae in undercooked beef*. In contrast to *T. solium*, these parasites contain a *scolex (head) with suckers, but no hooks*, and typical clinical manifestations are much milder, consisting of abdominal discomfort and weight loss.

➤ Diagnosis is via fecal examination for eggs and gravid proglottids.

HARDCORE REVIEW TABLES—INFECTIONS CAUSED BY WORMS (HELMINTHES) (TABLES 16-1 AND 16-2)

TABLE 16-1 Nematodes			
BUGS	**BUG POINTS**	**MOST COMMON PRESENTATION**	**HARDCORE MICROBIOLOGY**
Nematodes Acquired via Egg Ingestion			
Ascaris lumbricoides	• Intestinal nematode • Fecal–oral	Intestinal infection	*A. lumbricoides* eggs are visible in the feces of infected patients
Enterobius vermicularis	• Intestinal nematode • Fecal–oral	Pinworm infection • Intense night–time perianal itching	Found in children, diagnosis via "Scotch tape" test
Toxocara canis	• Blood and tissue nematode • Fecal–oral	Visceral larva migrans/toxocariasis • Fever • Diarrhea • Hepatitis • Chorioretinitis	Caused by dog roundworm larvae
Trichuris trichiura	• Intestinal nematode • Fecal–oral	Whipworm infection • Infection, abdominal complaints	Infection does not cause eosinophilia

(Continued)

TABLE 16-1	Nematodes (cont.)		
BUGS	**BUG POINTS**	**MOST COMMON PRESENTATION**	**HARDCORE MICROBIOLOGY**
Nematodes Acquired via Larvae Ingestion			
Dracunculus medinensis	• Blood and tissue nematode	Guinea worm infection • Nausea • Vomiting • Hives	Transmitted via ingestion of freshwater copepods in drinking water; female exposes her uterus to the environment to release microfilariae
Trichinella spiralis	• Intestinal nematode	Intestinal infection • Diarrhea • Abdominal pain • Fever	Follows the ingestion of encysted larvae typically found in raw pork
Nematodes Acquired via Larvae Skin Penetration			
Ancylostoma braziliense	• Blood and tissue nematode	Cutaneous larva migrans • Raised, itchy advancing rash	Larvae of dog hookworm; rash that advances called a "creeping eruption."
Ancylostoma duodenale *Necator americanus*	• Blood and tissue nematode • Intestinal nematode	Hookworm	Infection may result in clinical anemia Larvae travel to the lungs, where they are eventually coughed up and swallowed; cause iron-deficient anemia
Strongyloides stercoralis	• Intestinal nematode	Cryptococcal pneumonia, meningoencephalitis	Migrate to the lungs where they are coughed up and swallowed; autoinfective life-cycle; diagnosis by enterotest and fecal exam for larvae
Nematodes Acquired by Arthropod			
Loa loa	• Blood and tissue nematode	Loiasis • "Calabar swelling" • Granulomatous abscess formation • Conjunctiva damage	Transmitted to humans by day-biting *Chrysops* flies
Onchocerca volvulus	• Blood and tissue nematode	River blindness • Skin nodules • Developing rash of darkened pigmentation and dry scaly skin • Blindness	Spread to humans via the black fly, resulting in allergic response; microfilariae migration to the eye can lead to blindness, "lizard skin" rash
Wuchereria bancrofti	• Blood and tissue nematode	Elephantiasis, tropical pulmonary eosinophilia • Lymphatic backup with immense swelling and disfigurement	Spread via mosquito bite, nematode can accumulate in lymph nodes causing the lymphatic system to back up; serology exam for microfilaria done at night

TABLE 16-2	Platyhelminthes		
BUGS	**BUG POINTS**	**MOST COMMON PRESENTATION**	**HARDCORE MICROBIOLOGY**
Trematodes (Flukes)			
Clonorchis sinensis		Chinese liver fluke infection • Inflammation of the biliary tract	Transmitted via undercooked fish, may lead to obstructive jaundice resembling suppurative cholangitis
Paragonimus westermani		Lung fluke infection • Pulmonary inflammation	Follows ingestion of undercooked crustaceans (crab)
Schistosoma japonicum, mansoni, haematobium	• Blood fluke	Schistosomiasis/Katayama fever • Fever • Hives • Cough • Weight loss Possible development of: • Portal hypertension • Pulmonary hypertension • Inflammatory intestinal polyps	Mature within the freshwater snail, mate in hepatic portion of the portal venous system, eggs are laid in the bladder
Cestodes			
Diphyllobothrium latum		Fish tapeworm infection • Abdominal complications	May result in anemia caused by parasite-induced vitamin B_{12} deficiency
Echinococcus granulosus		Hydatid disease • Cyst formation in the lungs and liver	Found in dog feces; can enlarge, resulting in palpable liver masses and biliary obstruction; cysts may leak fluid, resulting in allergic reaction (anaphylaxis)
Taenia saginata		Beef tapeworm infection • Abdominal complaints	Passed by the ingestion of larvae in undercooked beef; scolex with suckers but no hooks
Taenia solium		Cysticercosis, Neurocysticercosis • Blindness • Seizures • Neurological deficits	Acquired by the ingestion of undercooked pork; hooks on scolex

CHAPTER 17

Hardcore Microbiology Concepts

Most of the questions you will face on Step 1 will be based on the microbial topics that have already been covered by this book. However, the board exam will also test you on certain concepts important in medical microbiology. Included in this chapter are laboratory techniques, enzymatic characteristics that help differentiate microorganisms in laboratory testing, hardcore microbial buzzwords, comparison figures of organisms by site of infection, and a plate series of testable photographs.

I. LABORATORY TECHNIQUES

The laboratory identification of organisms is based on a series of tests, including colonial morphology on agar, Gram stain, presence of spores, and biochemical tests including catalase and coagulase tests.

A. Microscopy

- **Visual examination**—Direct microscopic visual exam of feces, blood, urine, pus, CSF, sputum, or gastric lavage for organisms.
  - ○ **Fungi**
    - *Tinea*—Colorless, branching hyphae with cross-walls and anthroconidia.
    - *Mucor*—Irregular nonseptate hyphae with wide-angle branching.
    - *Aspergillus*—45-degree angle branching septate hyphae.
    - *Candida*—Pseudohyphae with budding yeast and germ tubes at 37°C.
    - *Cryptococcus*—Yeast with wide capsular halos and narrow-based unequal budding.
- **Light microscopy with special stains**
  - ○ *Ziehl-Nielsen*—Mycobacteria (acid-fast)
  - ○ *Silver methenasmine*—Stains chitin in cell walls of fungi
  - ○ *Giemsa*—Malaria, parasites (*Leishmania*), *Borrelia*, *Chlamydia*, trypanosomes
  - ○ *India ink*—*Cryptococcus neoformans*
  - ○ *Direct*—Parasites (stool)
  - ○ *Periodic acid Schiff* (PAS)—Glycogen and mucopolysaccharides
  - ○ *Gram*—CSF, bacteria
- **Electronmicroscopy**—Viruses

B. Culture

Amplifies organisms, which allows for detection by direct microscopy.
- **Liquid media**—Amplify the *direct number of organisms* present.
- **Solid media**—Produce *colonies* that allow for identification, susceptibility testing, and typing.
  - ○ Susceptibility testing is conducted by placing paper discs impregnated with antibiotics on agar inoculated with the test organism, and determining the degree of bacterial growth inhibition.
  - ○ Examples of specialized agar:
    - *Thayer-Martin*—N. gonorrhoeae
    - *Bordet-Gengou agar*—B. pertussis
    - *Chocolate agar*—H. influenzae
    - *Tellurite agar*—C. diphtheriae
    - *Charcoal yeast extract agar*—Legionella pneumophila
    - *Sabouraud's agar*—Fungi

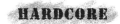

HARDCORE

The following bugs do not Gram stain and require different lab techniques: *Mycoplasma, Mycobacterium, Legionella pneumophilia, Chlamydia, Rickettsia,* and *Treponema*.

HARDCORE

Most human pathogens are "fastidious," requiring specific growth elements present in blood or serum, as well as the appropriate atmosphere (e.g., oxygen-free, oxygen present).

HARDCORE

Chocolate agar requires factors V, or NAD, as well as factor X, or hematin.

HARDCORE

Sabouraud's agar identifies *dimorphic fungi* by incubating cultures at 25°C in order to identify any branching hyphae, followed by increasing the temperature to 37°C to identify yeast cells. *Dimorphic fungi include*:
- *Sporothrix schenckii*
- *Candida albicans*
- *Cryptococcus*
- *Histoplasma*
- *Blastomyces*
- *Coccidioides*
- *Paracoccidioides*

- MacConkey's agar—**Lactose-fermenting enterics** including *Escherichia, Klebsiella, E. coli,* and *Enterobacter*
- Lowenstein-Jensen agar—M. tuberculosis

C. Serology Testing

Detects an *immune response to a pathogen*. Diagnosis is made by identifying rising or falling antibody levels in specimens more than a week apart, the presence of specific IgMs, or specific antigens.

- *Agglutination*—Detects bacterial capsular antigens in CSF.
- *Complement fixation.*
- *Virus neutralization.*
- *Radioimmunoassay (RIA)*—Used for the quantitation of any substance that can be labeled with a radioactive isotope including immunoglobulins or microbial capsules.
- *Enzyme-linked immunosorbent assay (ELISA)*—Measures antigens or antibodies.
- *Quellung reaction*—The capsule of encapsulated bacteria will swell in the presence of homologous antiserum. These organisms include:
  - *S. pneumonia*
  - *Neisseria meningitides*
  - *Haemophilus influenzae*
  - *Klebsiella pneumoniae*
- Fluorescent dyes—Antibodies specific to a pathogen are labeled with fluorescent marker. When viewed under ultraviolet light, bound antibody glows as a bright fluorescence.
  - RSV diagnosis

D. Molecular Techniques

- **Southern blotting**—A labeled DNA probe binds to the specimen and is detected by the activity of the labeled probe.
- **Nucleic acid amplification**—Amplifies pathogen target DNA or RNA, allowing detection.
  - *Polymerase chain reaction (PCR)*—After pathogen DNA is separated into single strands, specific primers and polymerase catalyses are added, resulting in the synthesis and amplification of new DNA.

II. MICROBIAL AND CLINICAL COMPARISON FIGURES (FIG. 17-1 TO FIG. 17-3)

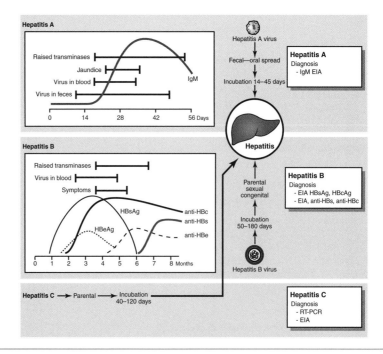

Figure 17–1 Comparison of the hepatitis viruses: hepatitis A, hepatitis B and hepatitis C.

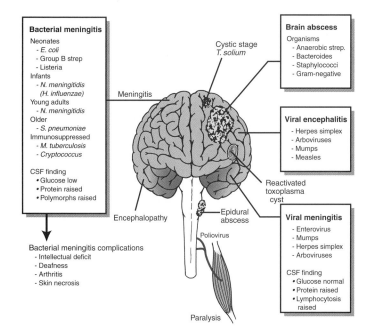

Bacterial meningitis

Neonates
- *E. coli*
- Group B strep
- Listeria

Infants
- *N. meningitidis*
  (*H. influenzae*)

Young adults
- *N. meningitidis*

Older
- *S. pneumoniae*

Immunosuppressed
- *M. tuberculosis*
- *Cryptococcus*

CSF finding
- Glucose low
- Protein raised
- Polymorphs raised

Bacterial meningitis complications
- Intellectual deficit
- Deafness
- Arthritis
- Skin necrosis

Meningitis

Encephalopathy

Cystic stage
T. solium

Brain abscess

Organisms
- Anaerobic strep.
- Bacteroides
- Staphylococci
- Gram-negative

Viral encephalitis
- Herpes simplex
- Arboviruses
- Mumps
- Measles

Reactivated
toxoplasma
cyst

Epidural
abscess

Poliovirus

Viral meningitis
- Enterovirus
- Mumps
- Herpes simplex
- Arboviruses

CSF finding
- Glucose normal
- Protein raised
- Lymphocytosis
  raised

Paralysis

Figure 17–2 Infections of the central nervous system—demographics and organisms.

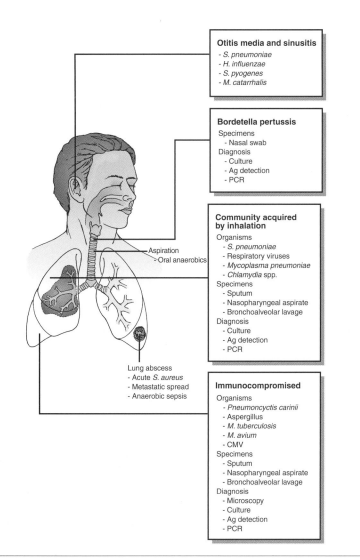

Otitis media and sinusitis
- *S. pneumoniae*
- *H. influenzae*
- *S. pyogenes*
- *M. catarrhalis*

Bordetella pertussis

Specimens
- Nasal swab

Diagnosis
- Culture
- Ag detection
- PCR

**Community acquired
by inhalation**

Organisms
- *S. pneumoniae*
- Respiratory viruses
- *Mycoplasma pneumoniae*
- *Chlamydia* spp.

Specimens
- Sputum
- Nasopharyngeal aspirate
- Bronchoalveolar lavage

Diagnosis
- Culture
- Ag detection
- PCR

Aspiration
Oral anaerobics

Lung abscess
- Acute *S. aureus*
- Metastatic spread
- Anaerobic sepsis

Immunocompromised

Organisms
- *Pneumocyctis carinii*
- Aspergillus
- *M. tuberculosis*
- *M. avium*
- CMV

Specimens
- Sputum
- Nasopharyngeal aspirate
- Bronchoalveolar lavage

Diagnosis
- Microscopy
- Culture
- Ag detection
- PCR

Figure 17–3 Common respiratory tract infections.

III. HARDCORE MICROBIOLOGY TABLES (TABLE 17-1 TO TABLE 17-3)

TABLE 17-1	Distinguishing Microbial Characteristics
ENZYME	**ASSOCIATED ORGANSISMS**
Catalase +	*Corynebacterium diphtheriae* *Listeria monocytogenes* *Mycobacterium avium-intracellulare* *Mycobacterium leprae* *Mycobacterium tuberculosis* *Propionibacterium acnes* *Staphylococcus aureus* *Staphylococcus epidermidis* *Staphylococcus saprophyticus* *Streptococcus viridans*
Catalase –	*Legionella pneumophila* *Streptococcus pneumoniae* *Streptococcus pyogenes*
Coagulase +	*Staphylococcus aureus*
Coagulase –	*Staphylococcus epidermidis* *Staphylococcus saprophyticus* *Streptococcus viridans*
Lactose fermenter	*Klebsiella pneumoniae* *Proteus mirabilis* *Serratia*
Non-lactose fermenter	*Haemophilus influenzae* *Pseudomonas aeruginosa* *Salmonella* *Shigella dysenteriae* *Yersinia pestis*
Oxidase +	*Campylobacter jejuni* *Eikenella corrodens* *Haemophilus influenzae* *Neisseria meningitides* and *gonorrhoeae* *Pseudomonas aeruginosa* *Vibrio cholerae*
Urease +	*Helicobacter pylori* *Proteus mirabilis*
Capsule	*Bacteroides fragilis* *Clostridium difficile* *Clostridium perfringens* *Enterococcus* *Francisella tularensis* *Haemophilus influenzae* *Legionella pneumophila* *Neisseria meningitides* and *gonorrhoeae* *Pasteurella multocida* *Serratia* *Staphylococcus epidermidis* *Staphylococcus saprophyticus* *Streptococcus agalactiae* *Streptococcus pneumoniae* *Streptococcus viridans* *Vibrio parahaemolyticus* *Yersina enterocolitica* *Yersinia pestis*

TABLE 17-2	Hardcore Microbial Buzzwords
BUZZWORD	**BUG**
Air-conditioning system	*Legionella pneumophila*
Anterior horn cell infection	Poliovirus
Argyll-Robertson pupil	*Treponema pallidum* (neurosyphilis)
Armadillos	*Mycobacterium leprae*
Atypical lymphocytes	Epstein-Barr virus
B$_{12}$ deficiency	*Diphyllobothrium latum*
Barking cough	Parainfluenza virus
Barrell-shaped eggs with bipolar plugs	*Trichuris trichiuria*
Beavers	*Giardia lambia*
Biliary obstruction	*Echinococcus granulosus*
Blue and green pigments	*Pseudomonas aeruginosa*
Blueberry muffin baby	Rubivirus

(Continued)

TABLE 17-2 Hardcore Microbial Buzzwords (cont.)

BUZZWORD	BUG
Break-bone fever	Dengue viruses
Bull's-eye-shaped nucleus	*Entamoeba histolytica*
Cat litter	*Toxoplasma gondii*
Cauliflower-like lesions	Human *Papillomavirus*
Chandelier sign	*Chlamydia trachomatis* *Neissera gonorrhea*
Chinese fried rice	*Bacilius cereus*
Chinese letters on microscope	*Corynebacterium diphtheriae*
"Christmas tree" distribution	Human herpesvirus 7
Cigar shaped	*Sporothrix schenckii*
Clue cells	*Gardnerella vaginalis*
Cold agglutinins	*Mycoplasma pneumoniae*
Comma shaped	*Vibrio cholerae*
Cough, conjunctivitis, coryza	Measles virus
Creeping eruption	*Ancylostoma braziliense*
Cruise ship outbreak	Noroviruses
Crustaceans (undercooked)	*Paragonimus westermani*
Current jelly sputum	*Klebsiella*
Dane particle	Hepatitis B
Dermatomal distribution	Varicella-zoster
Dishwater exudate	*Clostridium perfringens*
Exposes uterus in water	*Dracunculus medinensis*
Extending flagella appear as seagull wings	*Campylobacter jejuni*
Fishy vaginal discharge	*Gardnerella vaginalis*
Floppy baby	*Clostridium botulinum*
Flying saucer with silver stain	*Pneumocystis carinii*
Fried egg appearance	*Mycoplasma pneumoniae*
Ghon complex or focus	Tuberculosis
Golden-yellow pigment	*Staphylococcus aureus*
Honey-colored crusting on skin	*Streptococcus pyogenes*
"Honeymoon" cystitis	*Staphylococcus saprophyticus*
Human bites	*Eikenella corrodens*
Koilocytes	Human *Papillomavirus*
Koplik spots	Measles virus
Lizard skin rash	*Onchocerca volvulus*
Negri bodies	Rabies
Obstructive jaundice/cholangitis	*Clonorchis sinensis*
Pigeon droppings	*Cryptococcus neoformans*
Puppies	*Yersina enterocolitica*
Rabbits	*Francisella tularensis*
Rat urine	*Leptospira interrogans*
Red pigment	*Serratia*
Rice water stools	*Vibrio cholerae*
Rose gardeners disease	*Sporothrix schenckii*
Saftey-pin appearance on bipolar staining	*Yersinia pestis*
School of fish appearance	*Haemophilus ducreyi*
Scotch tape test	*Enterobius vermicularis*
Seafood	*Vibrio parahaemolyticus*
Strawberry cervix	*Trichomoniasis vaginalis*
Staghorn calculi	*Proteus mirabilis*
Sulfur granules	*Actinomyces israelii*
Syncytial effect	Respiratory syncytial virus
Tennis racquet appearance	*Clostridium tetani*
Trench mouth	*Fusobacterium*
Tumbling motility in 25°C broth	*Listeria monocytogenes*
White, clumpy, curd-like vaginal discharge	*Candida albicans*
Wool-sorter's disease	*Bacilius anthracis*

TABLE 17-3	Common Organisms by Site of Infection—All Demographics
Mouth	*Peptostreptococcus, Actinomyces, Treponema pallidum*
Skin and soft tissue	*Staphylococcus aureus, Streptococcus pyogenes, Staphylococcus epidermidis, Clostridium* spp.
Bone and joint	*Staphylococcus aureus, Streptococcus pyogenes, Neisseria gonorrhoeae*, Gram-negative bacilli
Abdominal	*E. coli, Proteus, Klebsiella, Enterococcus, Bacteroides* spp., *Clostridium* spp.
Urinary tract	*E. coli, Proteus, Klebsiella, Enterococcus* spp.
Upper respiratory tract	*Streptococcus pneumoniae, H. influenzae, Morazella catarrhalis, Streptococcus pyogenes*
Lower respiratory tract/community acquired	*Streptococcus pneumoniae, H. influenzae, Moraxella catarrhalis, Klebsiella, Legionella, Mycoplasma pneumoniae, Chlamydia pneumoniae*
Lower respiratory tract/hospital acquired	*Klebsiella, Pseudomonas aeruginosa, Staphylococcus aureus, Enterobacter, Serratia marcescens*
Meningitis	*Strepococcus pneumoniae, Neisseria meningitides, H. influenzae*, Group B *Streptococcus, E. coli, Listeria*

IV. HARDCORE MICROBIAL ORGANISMS—PLATES (FIG. 17-4 TO FIG. 17-15)

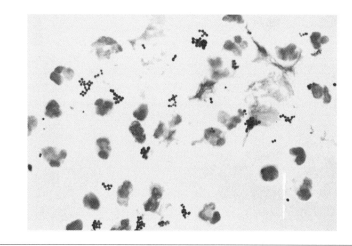

Figure 17–4 Gram stain of *Staphylococcus aureus* with polymorphonuclear neutrophils. *(Reprinted with permission from McClatchey KD. Clinical Laboratory Medicine, 2nd Edition. Philadelphia: Lippincott Williams & Wilkins, 2002).*

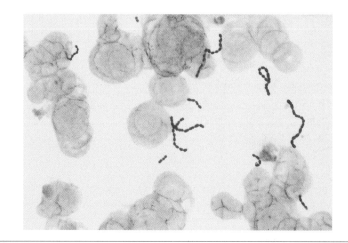

Figure 17–5 Gram stain of blood culture with streptococci. *(Reprinted with permission from McClatchey KD. Clinical Laboratory Medicine, 2nd Edition. Philadelphia: Lippincott Williams & Wilkins, 2002).*

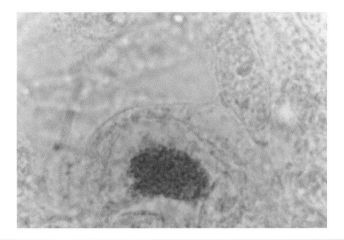

Figure 17–6 Chlamydial inclusion. *(Reprinted with permission from McClatchey KD. Clinical Laboratory Medicine, 2nd Edition. Philadelphia: Lippincott Williams & Wilkins, 2002).*

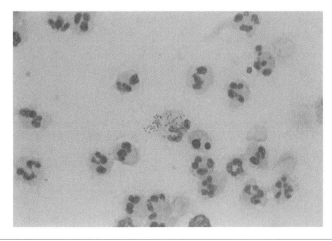

Figure 17–7 Gram stain of *Neisseria gonorrhoeae* in urethral exudates. *(Reprinted with permission from McClatchey KD. Clinical Laboratory Medicine, 2nd Edition. Philadelphia: Lippincott Williams & Wilkins, 2002).*

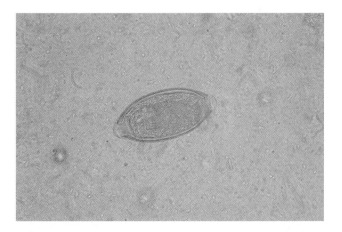

Figure 17–8 An egg of *T. trichiura*, showing the typical barrel shape, three-layer eggshell, and transparent bipolar plugs. *(Reprinted with permission from Sun, Tsieh. Parasitic Disorders: Pathology, Diagnosis, and Management, 2nd edition. Baltimore: Lippincott Williams & Wilkins, 1999).*

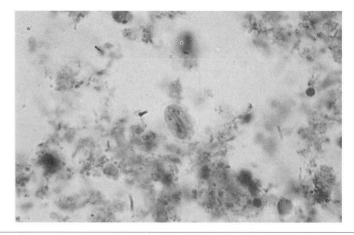

Figure 17–9 Cyst of *G. lamblia* in a fecal smear. *(Reprinted with permission from Sun, Tsieh. Parasitic Disorders: Pathology, Diagnosis, and Management, 2nd edition. Baltimore: Lippincott Williams & Wilkins, 1999).*

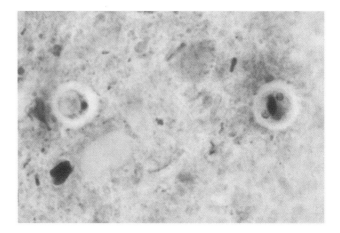

Figure 17–10 A cyst of *E. histolytica* (*right*) with three nuclei and a cigar-shaped chromatoidal body, and a precyst of the same species (*left*). *(Reprinted with permission from Sun, Tsieh. Parasitic Disorders: Pathology, Diagnosis, and Management, 2nd edition. Baltimore: Lippincott Williams & Wilkins, 1999).*

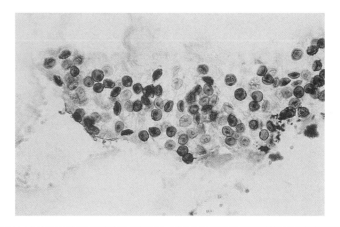

Figure 17–11 *Pneumocystis carinii* stained with silver stain. *(Reprinted with permission from McClatchey KD. Clinical Laboratory Medicine, 2nd Edition. Philadelphia: Lippincott Williams & Wilkins, 2002).*

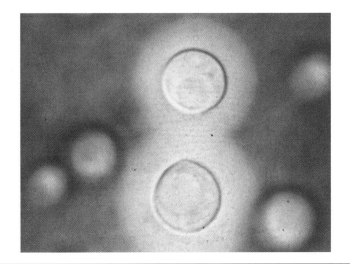

Figure 17–12 *Cryptococcus neoformans* (India ink preparation) shows halo effect around the yeast, caused by the large capsule. *(Reprinted with permission from Crapo JD, Glassroth J, Karlinsky JB. et al. Baum's Textbook of Pulmonary Diseases, 7th Edition. Philadelphia: Lippincott Williams & Wilkins, 2004).*

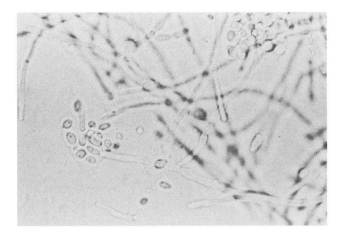

Figure 17–13 Branching hyphae of *Candida albicans. (Reprinted with permission from Sweet RL, Gibbs RS. Atlas of Infectious Diseases of the Female Genital Tract. Philadelphia: Lippincott Williams & Wilkins, 2005).*

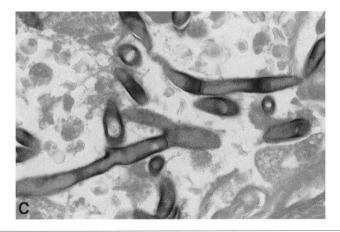

Figure 17–14 Lung tissue with invasive *Aspergillus* and characteristic true septae with 45-degree angle branching. *(Reprinted with permission from McClatchey KD. Clinical Laboratory Medicine, 2nd Edition. Philadelphia: Lippincott Williams & Wilkins, 2002).*

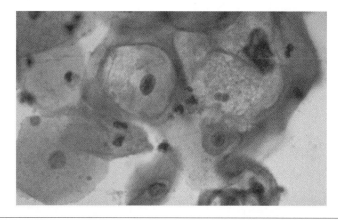

Figure 17–15 Human *Papillomavirus*-induced condylomatous infection: cervical smear contains characteristic koilocytes, with a perinuclear halo and a wrinkled nucleus that contains viral particles. *(Reprinted with permission from Rubin E and Farber JL. Pathology, 3rd Edition. Philadelphia: Lippincott Williams & Wilkins, 1999).*

CHAPTER 18

Immunology: The Players

The immune system is comprised of a group of cells and substances found within the body that are capable of defending us against infections, cancer, and compounds foreign to the human body. Most of the major players in the immune system are cells derived from precursors in the bone marrow that circulate in the blood and enter tissues where needed. These cells form from stem cells that differentiate into mature cells based on type of cellular lineage and growth factors present.

I. MYELOID LINEAGE

Myeloid lineage cells are derived from the granulocyte—monocyte common precursor. These cells are capable of differentiating into cells in the myeloid series based on the presence of "growth" or "colony-stimulating" factors (Fig. 18-1).

- **Granulocytes:**
    - Neutrophils
    - Eosinophils
    - Basophils
    - Mast cells
- **Mononuclear cells:**
    - Monocytes
    - Macrophages
- **Megakaryocytes**
- **Dendritic cells**

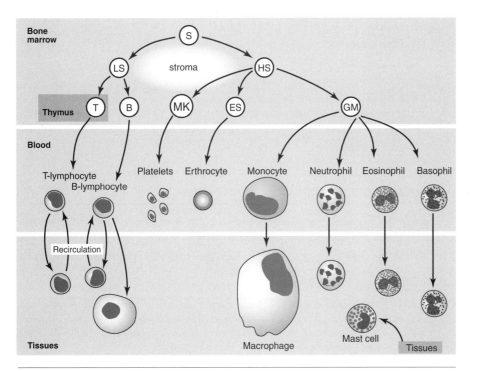

Figure 18–1 Cellular differentiation within the immune system. (B, bone marrow-derived lymphocyte; ES, erythroid stem cell; GM, granulocyte—monocyte; HS, hemopoietic stem cell; LS, lymphoid stem cell; MK, megakaryocyte; S, stem cel; T, thymus-derived lymphocyte.)

A. Granulocytes

Granulocytes are also known as **polymorphonuclear leukocytes**.

- **Neutrophils**—The most abundant of the circulating polymorphonuclear cells.
  - Active phagocytes.
  - Highly motile.
  - Possess receptors for antibodies and complement on their surface.
  - Azurophilic granules contain *myeloperoxidase* (MPO), which produces hypochlorous acid.
- **Eosinophils**—These granulocytes are responsible for combating infection by *parasites* in the body. They make up 1.5% of the total WBC count.
  - Eosinophil *granules are bright yellow-red or orange and contain histamine* and other chemicals toxic to parasites.
  - They play a role in the allergic response (*asthma and serum sickness*).
- **Basophils**—The least common granulocyte, representing about 1% of circulating leukocytes.
  - Store histamine in their granules.
  - Appear in specific types of inflammatory response (allergic symptoms).
  - Have protein receptors on their cell surface that bind IgE antibody.
- **Mast cells**—A resident cell of connective tissue that contains many granules rich in *histamine and heparin*. The two types of mast cells include connective tissue mast cells and mucosal mast cells.
  - Play an important role in *allergy and anaphylaxis*, and are involved in wound healing and defense against pathogens.
  - Express a high-affinity receptor for *IgE*.
  - A generalized degranulation of mast cells may result in vasodilatation and, if severe enough, life-threatening *shock* (anaphylaxis).

B. Mononuclear Cells

Mononuclear cells give rise to *monocytes*, which develop into macrophages after migrating into tissues.

- **Macrophages (MACs)**—Found in tissues and serous cavities (e.g., pleura and peritoneum), these cells phagocyze pathogens. MACs are derived from the bone marrow and exist in two forms:

  1. **Free**—Monocytes, which are the largest nuceloid cells in the blood.
  2. **Fixed to tissue**—Found in most tissues.

  MACs are attracted to sites of inflammation by circulating cytokines (C5a), and have three main functions:

  1. Phagocytosis.
  2. Antigen presentation—MACs utilize MHC class II proteins.
  3. Cytokine production—IL-1 and TNF-alpha.

- **Dendritic cells**—Dendritic cells are present in low frequency in tissues that are in contact with the environment, including the skin (where they are often called **Langerhans cells**), nose, lungs, stomach, and intestines. These cells act as antigen-presenting cells by taking up antigens and migrating to T-cell areas within lymph nodes or the spleen.

II. LYMPHOID LINEAGE

Lymphoid stem cells are capable of differentiating into B- and T-cells. Unlike other hematopoetic cells, lymphocytes do not divide (normally) unless stimulated by exposure to antigens and growth factors.

A. B-Cells

B-lymphocytes produce *antibodies* (Abs), which are glycoproteins receptors consisting of two identical *heavy chains* and two identical *light chains* connected by interchain disulfide bonds. Antibodies are a fundamental component of the humoral element of adaptive immunity (Fig. 18-2).

Important components of the antibody structure include:

- **Carboxyl terminal region** of the heavy and light chains comprise the *constant* part of the chain.
- **Amino terminal region** of the heavy and light chains comprise the *variable* part of the chains.

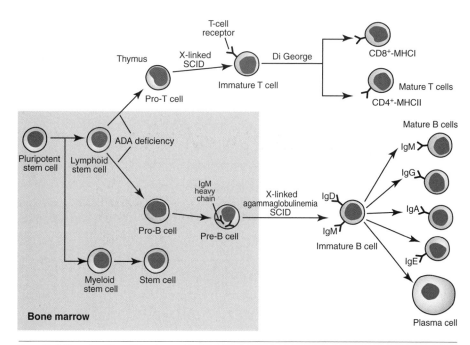

Figure 18–2 Maturation of B- and T-lymphocytes. After hemopoietic stem cells give rise to progenitor cells, the latter enter either the B-cell (bone marrow) or T-cell (thymus) developmental pathway. In the thymus, CD4 and CD8 are transiently expressed on immature T-cells. Maturation to CD4+ or CD8+ T-cells is determined by the interaction of CD4 with MHC class II or of CD8 with MHC class I molecules on thymic stromal cells. In the bone marrow, the interaction of progenitor B-cells with stromal cells yields pre-B—cells. After leaving the bone marrow, pre-B—cells differentiate into mature, Ig-specific B-cells and eventually Ig-secreting plasma cells. Immunodeficiencies affect these pathways. Common examples include Di George syndrome, ADA deficiency, and X-linked agammaglobulinemia.

In the laboratory, *papain* (a proteolytic enzyme) is used to split an antibody into three parts (Fig. 18-3):

- Two identical *Fab fragments*
  ○ Each fragment with one site capable of binding antigen.
  ○ Composed of both heavy and light chains.
- One *Fc fragment*
  ○ Does not bind antigens.
  ○ Composed of *only heavy chains*.

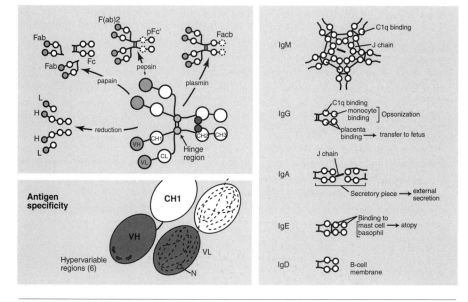

Figure 18–3 Antibody structure and function.

Similarly, *pepsin* (another proteolytic enzyme) splits the antibody but at a different site, resulting in two fragments:

- Fc fragment
- F(ab)2
  - Similar to the parent molecule, it is capable of binding two antigens.

Variability of Antibodies

- **Isotypes**—Differences in the constant region
  - The heavy-chain constant region is one of five different types that define the immunoglobulin isotypic variants: *IgM, IgA, IgD, IgG, IgE*.
  - Similarly, the light-chain constant regions form isotypic variants for each Ig molecule composed of either kappa (κ)-type or lambda (λ)-, but never both.
  - A single gene encodes each constant region.
- **Variable Region**—The gene cluster that encodes for the light chains (κ or λ) and the heavy chains contains:
  - A collection of ~50 variable region (V) genes.
  - ~5 Joining (J) genes.
  - Only the heavy chains contain a section of ~25 highly variable (D) genes.

Both the κ or λ light-chain variable regions are encoded by two different gene segments. One of the V segments joins with one of the J segments from each light-chain variable region, resulting in VλJλ and VκJκ. Each segment subsequently binds to a constant (C) segment, resulting in VJC.

- Antibody classes
  - IgM
    - Marker of a primary infection, this is the first antibody to be secreted by newly activated naïve B-cells.
    - In serum, this immunoglobulin forms pentamers by the union of the monomeric IgM constant region via J chains.
  - IgA
    - *Plasma IgA* is monomeric, while *secretary IgA* is a dimer secreted in saliva, tears, nasal fluid, sweat, colostrums, lung, genitourinary tract, and gastrointestinal tract.
    - In mucous, secretory IgA binds soluble antigens and blocks their entrance into the body.
  - IgD
    - Most IgD molecules are present in conjunction with IgM on the surface of B-cells, acting together to facilitate B-cell activation or suppression.
  - IgG
    - IgG is the *most abundant Ig*.
    - IgG is the main immunoglobulin synthesized during the secondary response and is capable of activating the classical complement pathway, as well as inducing opsonization.
  - IgE
    - IgE plays an important role in allergic reactions and in some parasitic infections.
    - Binds with high affinity receptors onto mast cells. If an allergen binds with this abnormal immunoglobulin, it results in mast cell degranulation and the release of inflammatory mediators and vasoactive compounds. If this occurs systemically, severe hypotension and shock may ensue.
- Immunoglobulin epitopes—The epitope is the part of the antigen recognized by an antigen receptor.
  - **Allotype** (polymorphic)—May be on the light or heavy chain; this epitope differs among members of the *same species*.
  - **Idiotype**—Determined by the antigen-binding site, the idiotype is *unique for a given antigen*.
  - **Isotype**—Common to a *single class of immunoglobulin* (IgA-IgE), determined by the heavy chain.

B. T-Cells

T-lymphocytes differentiate in the thymus and are specialized for operation *against cells containing intracellular organisms* (Fig. 18-4). These lymphocytes use T-cell receptors (TCRs) that recognize antigens and cell surface markers called *major histocompatibility complex (MHC)* on the cell surface of host cells.

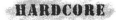

One Ig pentamer can bind up to 20 antigens, and therefore is considered a very effective bacterial agglutinator and complement activator.

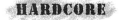

Aggregated IgA is capable of activating phagocytic cells and the alternative complement pathway.

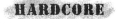

Antigen bound with at least two IgG molecules activates the complement cascade by binding C1q.

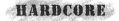

The phagocytic activity of PMNs and macrophages is greatly enhanced when bacteria are coated with IgG.

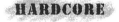

IgG is the only Ig capable of crossing the placenta, and thus provides an important line of defense for the first few months of an infant's life.

HARDCORE

Allotype testing is used in paternity cases because the epitopes vary among members of the human species.

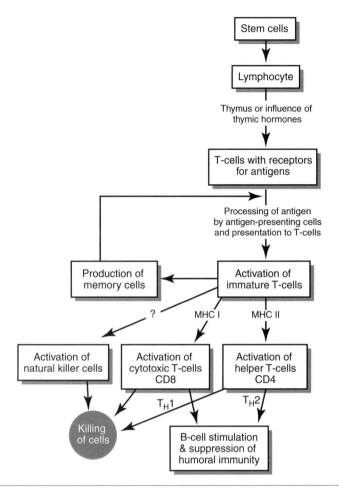

Figure 18–4 Overview of important T-cell actions.

- **T-cell receptors**—Consists of α and β chains, and the encoding of the receptor is similar to that of antibodies. The variable region is formed by random rearrangement of clusters of V, D (only for β chains), and J segments to form V+-DJ for each chain.

- **Helper T-cells**—Act in antibody and cell-mediated responses. These cells *have CD4 surface marker and bind MHC class II on antigen-presenting cells*. Helper T-cells can be further differentiated based on the cytokines secreted and which component of the adaptive immune response they act on (Fig. 18-5).

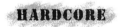 **HARDCORE**

The CD3 complex connects to TCR and functions as a transducer following antigen binding.

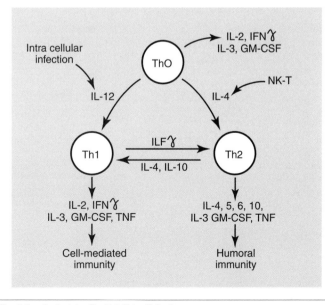

Figure 18–5 Differentiation of naïve helper T-cell into Th1 or Th2 cells.

○ **Th1 cells**—Involved in cell-mediated immunity, these cells produce *gamma-interferon and IL-2, which activates MACs and cytotoxic T-cells*. Th1 cells are important for eliminating intracellular infections.

○ **Th2 cells**—Involved in antibody-mediated immunity, these cells *produce IL-4 and IL-5*. Th2 cells help B-cells make antibodies that target foreign bodies, capsule pathogens, and toxins.

- **Cytotoxic T-cells**—These cells have *CD8 surface markers* and kill target cells following recognition of *foreign peptide-MHC class I molecules* on the target cell membrane.

  ○ These cells kill virus-infected cells.

  ○ T-cells preferentially kill by secreting perforins and granzymes that activate target cells to undergo apoptosis (programmed cell death). This is a calcium-dependent process.

III. CELL SURFACE MARKERS

Cell surface molecules are vital for normal cellular interaction with components of the immune system.

A. Major Histocompatibility Complex (MHC)

These molecules act as cell surface markers that *allow infected cells to signal both cytotoxic T-cells and helper T-cells*. Additionally, the ability of T-cells to recognize antigens is dependent on the association of antigens with MHC. Clinically, these interactions are important for successful organ transplants and in treating autoimmune disorders. There are two main classes of MHC:

- **Class I**—Exists on *all nucleated cells*.
  ○ Encoded by HLA-A, B, C.
  ○ Molecule consists of *one polypeptide*, with beta2-microglobulin.
- **Class II**—Expressed on *antigen-presenting cells* (MACs, B-cells, dendritic cells).
  ○ Encoded by HLA-DR, DQ, DP.
  ○ Molecule consists of *two polypeptides*, one alpha and one beta chain.

B. Cluster of Differentiation (CD)

A cluster of differentiation (CD) consists of a cluster of monoclonal cells that react with the same polypeptide. There are currently over 250 CD numbers assigned, but for boards you should be familiar with those listed in Table 18-1.

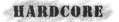

Class II MHC are the main determinants of organ rejection.

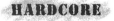

Superantigens are certain molecules, including specific viruses and staphylococcal enterotoxins, which have the ability to cross-link both the variable domain of the TCR beta chain and the MHC II (not CD4) *outside* of the peptide-binding site. This induces a *massive T-cell activation* with excessive and dangerous over production of cytokines.

TABLE 18-1	**Common Clusters of Differentiation and their Functions**	
CD NUMBER	**EXPRESSION**	**FUNCTION**
CD1	Interdigitating dendritic cells	Presents glycolipids and other nonpeptide antigens to T-cells
CD3	T-cells	Transduces elements of the T-cell receptor
CD4	T-helpers, MACs, monocytes	MHC class II, HIV receptor
CD5	T- and B-lymphocytes	Involved in Ag receptor signaling
CD8	T-cytotoxic	MHC class I
CD14	Granulocytes, MACs, monocytes	LPS/LBS complex receptor
CD19	B-lymphocytes, dendritic cells	Part of B-cell Ag receptor complex
CD20	B-lymphocytes	Intracellular signals
CD21	B-lymphocytes, dendritic cells	Receptor for C3d and Epstein-Barr virus, part of B-cell Ag receptor complex
CD34	Progenitors	Adhesion molecule, stem cell marker
CD56	Nucleated cells	Important for NK cell recognition

CHAPTER 19

Immunology: The Game

In general, the immune system recognizes and sorts "self" matter from nonself matter. Nonself is considered anything different from a person's own molecular composition. The most common form of nonself matter is micro-organisms, but may also include substances such as drugs, mutated cancer cells, or a food (e.g., peanuts).

- The immune system acts through a number of simple and complex mechanisms to keep the human body "clean" by attempting to remove all foreign objects. When reading this chapter, keep in mind that *bacterial infection* results in a host **humoral immune response** causing a mobilization of B-cells, polymorphnuclear leukocytes (PMNs), and Th2 cells; while *viruses, fungi, mycobacteria, protozoa, parasites, and neoplasms* result in a **cell-mediated immune response** mediated by T-cells and macrophages.

I. INITIAL DEFENSIVE BARRIERS

Before any nonself material is recognized and processed, it must first penetrate the body. These barriers act as the first line of defense:

- **Surface barriers:** Intact skin is impermeable to most microorganisms.
- **Mucous membranes:** Enzymes (in saliva and tears), mucus, acid (stomach low pH).
- **Microbial antagonism:** The natural microbial flora of a person may fend off potential pathogenic microbes.

If an organism penetrates the body, then there are two main types of immune responses that can be activated: *the natural or acquired immune response* (Table 19-1).

TABLE 19-1	Overview of Important Cytokines and their Functions	
CYTOKINE	**SOURCE**	**FUNCTION**
IL-1	Monocyte macrophage NK cell, B-cell	• Costimulates T-cell activation through increased production of IL-2 • Induces IL-1, 6, 8, TNFα, GM-CSF by macrophages • NK cell cytotoxicity • Enhances B-cell proliferation and maturation proinflammatory • Induces fever
IL-2	Th1	• Induces proliferation of T- and B-cells • Enhances tumor cell killing and bacteria by monocytes and macrophages
IL-3	T-cells, NK cell, mast cell	• Induces growth and differentiation of hematopoetic precursors • Stimulates mast cell growth
IL-4	Th2, NK cell	• Induces Th2 cells • Stimulates proliferation/activation of B-cells • Induces immunoglobulin switch to IgG and IgE
IL-5	Th2, mast cell	• Induces proliferation of eosinophils • Stimulates switch to IgA
IL-6	Th2, monocyte	• Differentiation of myeloid stem cells and B-cells into plasma cells • Enhances T-cell proliferation
IL-8	Monocyte	• Mediates chemotaxis and activates neutrophils
IL-10	Th, B-cell, monocyte	• Inhibits IL-2 and Th1 cells • Inhibits Th1 cell differentiation and T-cell proliferation • Enhances B-cell differentiation

(Continued)

TABLE 19-1	Overview of Important Cytokines and their Functions (cont.)	
CYTOKINE	**SOURCE**	**FUNCTION**
IL-12	Monocyte	• Th1 differentiation • Enhances NK and CD8 T cytotoxicity
TNFα	Th, monocyte, mast cell, NK cell, B-cell	• Tumor cytotoxicity • Stimulates cytokine secretion • Antiviral • Cancer cachexia
IFNα	Leukocyte	• Inhibits viral replication • Enhances MHC class I
IFN β	Fibroblast	• Inhibits viral replication • Enhances MHC class I
IFN γ	Th1, NK cell	• Inhibits viral replication • Enhances MHC class I and II • Inhibits proliferation of Th2
GM-CSF	Th, endothelium, fibroblast, mast cell	• Stimulates growth of progenitors of monocytes, neutrophils, eosinophils, and basophils • Activates macrophages
G-CSF	Fibroblast endothelium	• Stimulates growth of neutrophil progenitors
M-CSF	Fibroblast, endothelium, epithelium	• Stimulates growth of monocyte progenitors
TGF β	B-cell, macrophage, mast cell	• Proinflammatory

II. NATURAL (INNATE) IMMUNE RESPONSE

HARDCORE

Lack of innate immune response is seen clinically in *chronic granulomatous disease*, resulting in defective killing of phagocytosed microorganisms.

The natural or innate response (Fig. 19-1) is a nonspecific system that *lacks immunologic memory*, and therefore this immune response will be unchanged regardless of how frequently an antigen is encountered.

A. Types of Innate Immune Responses

Phagocytosis

Phagocytosis is a three-step process that involves enclosing a target antigen into an intracellular phagosome, fusing it with cytoplasmic granules, and killing it with an oxidative burst. Types of cells involved in phagocytosis include:

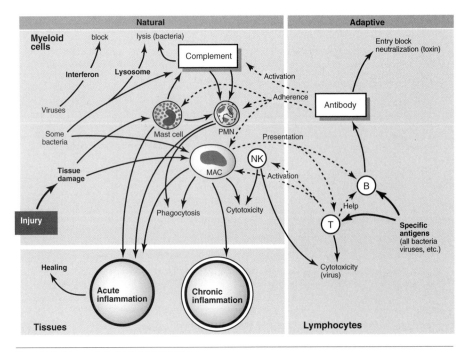

Figure 19–1 Natural and adaptive immune responses.

- **Macrophages:**
  - ○ Macrophages recognize sugar moieties present on the outer layers of micro-organisms, including:
    - ▪ A gram-negative outer layer composed of *lipopolysaccharides (LPS)*.
    - ▪ A gram-positive *teichoic acid cell wall*. This is recognized by the macrophage pattern recognition receptor, which activates a signal cascade initiating the phagocytosis of the micro-organisms and the up-regulation proinflammatory genes.
  - ○ Important tissues that contain MACs include:
    - ▪ **Lung**—Alveolar macrophages
    - ▪ **Liver**—Kupffer cells
    - ▪ **Spleen sinusoids**—RES cells
    - ▪ **Lymph node medullary sinuses**—Dendritic cells
    - ▪ Throughout **basement membranes of blood vessels**
    - ▪ **Kidney**—Mesangial cells
    - ▪ **Skin**—Langerhans cells
    - ▪ **Brain**—Microglial cells
    - ▪ **Bone**—Osteoclasts
    - ▪ **Connective tissue**—Schistocytes, giant cells, or epithelioid cells
- **Polymorphonuclear cells/neutrophils**—Contain two main types of granules:
  - ○ **Primary azurophilic granules**
    - ▪ Myeloperoxidases
    - ▪ Defensins
    - ▪ Cathepsin G
  - ○ **Secondary specific granules**:
    - ▪ Lactoferrin
    - ▪ Lysozyme

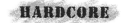

Inside a macrophage phagolysosome, an organism is attacked by a multitude of deadly oxidative radicals including toxic superoxide anion, hydroxyl radicals, hypochlorous acid, nitric oxide, antimicrobial cationic proteins and peptides, and lysozymes.

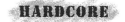

Eosinophils are only weakly phagocytic and, on activation, probably kill parasites mainly by releasing cationic proteins and reactive oxygen metabolites into the extracellular fluid.

Inflammatory Mediators

Inflammatory mediators are released by basophils, mast cells, and eosinophils.

- **Interleukin(IL)-1, IL-6, tumor necrosis factor (TNF)**
  - ○ *Produce fever*. Many microorganisms have adapted for optimal growth at body temperature; thus, an increase in temperature can partially inhibit growth.
  - ○ Also increase leukocyte adherence, act as procoagulants, and induce fibroblast proliferation.
- **Interferon**—These proteins place uninfected cells in an antiviral state and induce the production of proteins that inhibit viral protein synthesis.
  - ○ Induces activity of intracellular DNAses and RNAses that enzymatically cut strands of viral DNA or mRNA particles.
  - ○ Also stimulates NKC phagocytic activity.

Natural Killer Cells

Natural killer cells (NKCs) cause the nonspecific destruction of *virus-infected and tumor malignant cells* by secreting cytokines and Fas-Fas ligand binding apoptosis. NKC receptors include:

- **Killer-activating receptors**—Recognize a number of different molecules that are present on the surface of all nucleated cells. If these receptors are occupied, a signal is sent to the NKC to destroy the cell.
  - ○ In normal cells, this signal is hampered by an inhibitory signal sent by the killer-inhibitory receptor after recognition of MHC I molecules.
  - ○ If a cell is infected by a microorganism or if the cell transforms to a malignant cell, MHC I molecules are lost, informing the NKCs to destroy the cell.
  - ○ NKCs are mobilized by IL-12 and gamma-interferon cytokines.
- **NKC Fc receptors**—Bind IgG (FcNKCR).
  - ○ These receptors link natural killer cells to IgG-coated target cells. These cells are then killed by antibody-dependent cellular cytotoxicity (acquired immunity).

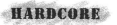

In cancer patients, IL-1 and TNF-alpha mediate tumor-induced cachexia by increasing catabolism of proteins and fat.

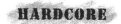

All host nucleated cells have MHC class I and CD56 molecules on their surface for NKC recognition.

Complement Cascade

The complement system is a group of serum proteins that produce effector molecules involved in *inflammation (C3a, C5a), phagocytosis (C3b), and cell lysis (C5b-9)*. Together, these processes make up an important defense against micro-organisms, particularly *gram-negative bacteria*.

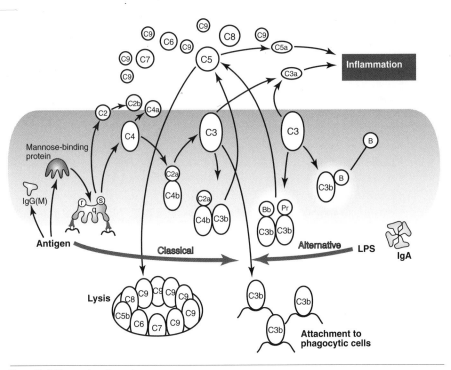

Figure 19–2 The complement cascade.

The complement cascade is activated by three different mechanisms (Fig. 19-2):

1. *Classical pathway*—Antibody–antigen complex (acquired immune response).

   • This pathway is initiated by the binding of specific IgG or IgM antibody to surface antigens, which are subsequently recognized by a *calcium-dependent* C1 component.

   • Activated C1 attacks C2 and C4.

   • Attacked C2 splits into small (C2b) and large (C2a) fragments, while C4 also splits into small (C4a) and large (C4b) fragments.

   • C4b and C2a join and attach to the antigen–antibody complex, forming *C3 convertase*.

   • C3 convertase splits C3 into small (C3a) and large (C3b) fragments. Some C3b is deposited on the membrane, acting as an attachment site for phagocytic polymorphs and MACs, while the rest of the C3b remains associated with C4b and C2a, forming *C5 convertase*.

   • C5 convertase splits C5 into C5a (small), which combines with C3a to promote the inflammatory response (acts on mast cells, polymorphs, and smooth muscle); and C5b (large), which initiates the assembly of C6-9 and the membrane attack complex.

2. *Alternative pathway*—Activated by toxins, microbial-cell walls, and IgA (innate immune response).

   • This pathway is initiated by a variety of toxins and polysaccharides and some antibodies (IgA). In the absence of antibodies, molecules that are carbohydrate or lipid in nature, including microbial mannose and liposaccharides (LPS), can activate the complement system. This pathway is *not dependent* on calcium ions, C1, C2, or C4 components (the classical pathway *is dependent* on these components).

   • The alternative pathway initiates C3 conversion with bacterial products or IgA, resulting in the complex of factor B with C3b.

   • Next, factor D acts on the C3b-B complex, producing the active *convertase C3bBb*.

   • Properdin stabilizes the C3b-B complex, allowing further C3 conversion and the subsequent activation of *C5 convertase*. This pathway then follows the assembly of the membrane attack complex.

3. *Lytic pathway*—Results in direct lysis of bacterial cell membranes, resulting in leakage of intracellular components and cell death.

   • Initiated by the *splitting of C5 by a convertase* (either *classical*: C3b-C2a-C4b; or *alternative*: C3b-factor Bb-properdin).

   • Serum components C6–C8 merge with ten or more molecules of C9, creating the *membrane attack complex* that inserts into cell membranes of bacteria and results in cell lysis.

Acute-Phase Response

The acute-phase response is an innate body defense seen during acute illnesses. Either the presence of foreign bodies (bacteria) within the body or tissue injury provokes a protective inflammatory response (acute inflammation), resulting in:

- Increased blood flow.
- Increased capillary permeability at the focus of injury, which allows lymphatic blood cells and serum components to gain access to the compromised tissue.

This response is characterized clinically by the presence of swelling, redness, warmth, and pain at the site of infection. The first cells to arrive at the site of injury (*neutrophils and macrophages*) secrete a number of protein molecules, called *cytokines*, into the bloodstream that function to recruit other cells and stop an impending invasion (Fig. 19-3 and Table 19-1). The most important include:

- **IL-1**
  - ○ Secreted by macrophages.
  - ○ Activates T- and B-lymphocytes, neutrophils, and fibroblasts.
- **IL-6**
  - ○ Secreted by T-cells and macrophages.
  - ○ Induces the productions of acute-phase proteins by the liver.
- **TNF-alpha**
  - ○ Released by macrophages.
  - ○ Also known as *cachectin*.
  - ○ Stimulates the acute-phase response in the liver.

These circulating cytokines cause a response in multiple organs:

1. **Liver**—Responds to circulating cytokines (IL-6) by producing a large number of proteins (*acute-phase proteins*). These proteins are produced to both micro-organism invasion and other forms of tissue injury:

   - **C-reactive protein**
     - ○ A pentameric globulin whose levels rise dramatically within hours of tissue damage or infection.
     - ○ Binds phosphorylcholine found on the surface of many bacteria, fixes complement, and promotes phagocytosis.
     - ○ Induces the release of cytokines and tissue factor in monocytes.

   - **Mannose-binding protein**
     - ○ Binds to the surface of bacteria and enhances the activation of the complement alternative pathway.

HARDCORE

IL-1 is an endogenous pyrogen, which acts on the hypothalamus to cause the fever seen in infections. IL-6 is the chief stimulator of the production of most acute-phase proteins by the liver.

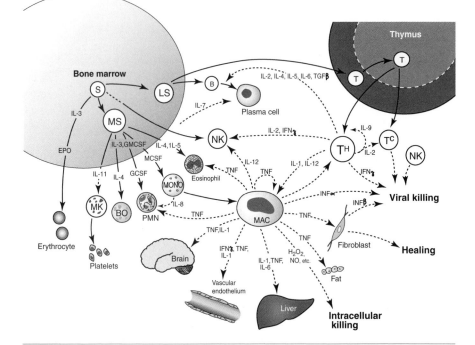

Figure 19–3 Cytokine overview.

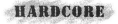

- **Coagulation factors**—Fibrinogen, prothrombin, factor VIII, von Willebrand factor, plasminogen
- **Complement factors**

2. **Bone Marrow**—Stimulates the production of colony-stimulating factor (CSF), resulting in leukocytosis.

3. **Hypothalamus**—Peripheral cytokines can act on the hypothalamus to up-regulate the body temperature, causing fever.

4. **Fat and Muscle**—Cytokines increase the mobilization of energy reserves to raise body temperature.

5. **T-cell mobilization**—T-cells mediate a variety of reactions, including:

- Cytotoxic destruction of virus-infected cells and bacteria.
- Activation of macrophages.
- Delayed hypersensitivity.
- Also help B-cells to produce antibody against many antigens.

6. **B-cell mobilization**—The production of IL-4 and IL-5 by activated helper T-cells *turns on* or activates antibody-producing B-cells. Immunoglobulins protect against organisms by several mechanisms, including:

- Neutralizing toxins.
- Lysis of bacteria in the presence of complement.
- Opsonization of bacteria facilitates phagocytosis.
- Interfering with the adherence of bacteria and viruses to cell surfaces.

III. ADAPTIVE IMMUNITY

Adaptive immunity is comprised of *cellular and humoral elements* that respond to a *specific stimulus* (Fig. 19-4). This immunity results in the development of host memory, allowing faster recognition and more intense robust immune response the next time that organism is encountered (secondary response).

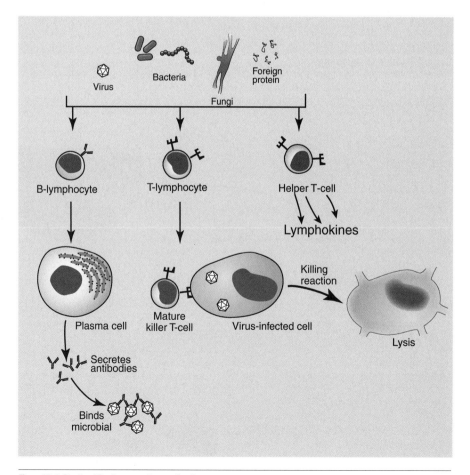

Figure 19–4 B-cell and T-cell response to nonself antigens.

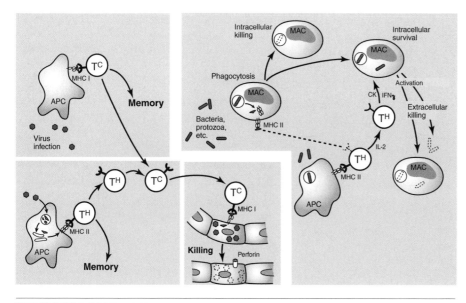

Figure 19–5 Cell-mediated immune response.

A. Cell-Mediated Immunity

Cell-mediated immunity (CMI) is an immune response involving the activation of macrophages, the production of antigen-specific cytotoxic T-lymphocytes, and the release of various cytokines in response to an antigen (Fig. 19-5).

1. A bacterium enters the body and is ingested by a macrophage.

2. The bacterium is broken down and its fragments, called *antigens* or *epitopes*, are expressed on the surface of the macrophage in association with *class II MHC* proteins.

3. Antigens and class II MHC proteins interact with antigen-specific receptors on the surface of CD4 T-lymphocytes.

4. Interleukins IL-1 and IL-2 cause helper T-cell activation and clonal proliferation of this antigen-specific helper T-cell.

5. Together, T-lymphocytes and macrophages destroy the offending agent.

6. In virus-infected cells or cells infected with intracellular pathogens, the infected cells express their epitope with *class I MHC protein*. A cytotoxic T-cell will kill any cell whose surface they recognize as having the same combination of class I MHC antigen plus virus.

B. Humoral-Mediated Immunity

Humoral immunity denotes antibody-mediated immune responses. Humoral immunity is directed at *toxin-inducing disease, infections by micro-organisms with polysaccharide capsules (pneumococci, meningococci, H. influenzae), and certain viral infections*. This type of adaptive immunity relies primarily on the actions of *antibodies* to act against infectious agents and their products. Antibodies function by three important mechanisms:

1. **Neutralize toxins and viruses**—Bind and prevent adherence.

2. **Opsonize organism**—Cause the improved phagocytosis of organisms.

3. **Complement activation**—Activate complement-enhancing opsonization and lysis.

Immunoglobulins are produced only as a result of stimulation by foreign antigens in a process known as the *antibody response*, which consists of two different responses. The *primary response* occurs the first time a specific antigen interacts with the immune system, and the *secondary response* results following any subsequent antigen run-ins.

• **Primary response**—The first time an antigen is encountered (Fig. 19-6).

1. An antigen is encountered and processed by an APC. Fragments of the Ag are presented along with MHC class II proteins to a helper T-cell within the T-area of a lymph node.

2. This helper T-cell produces *IL-2, IL-4, and IL-5,* which activate a B-cell capable of producing Abs specific for that Ag.

3. The activated B-cell proliferates and differentiates, forming multiple *plasma cells* that secrete huge numbers of immunoglobulins, which seek out and bind to specific antigens present infecting the host.

4. The first antibodies to appear during the primary response are *IgM*, followed by IgG or IgA.

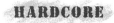

During the primary response, antibodies are detected after 7 to 10 days of B-cell proliferation. This is called a "lag period," and is considerably longer than the lag period of the secondary response (3 to 5 days).

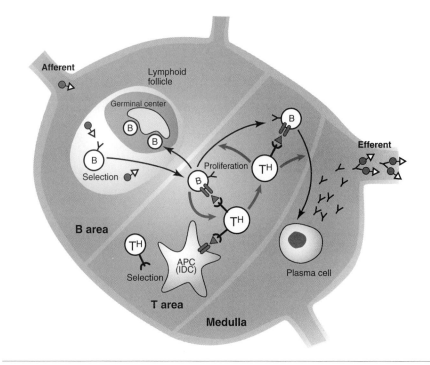

Figure 19–6 Primary antibody response.

- **Secondary response**—Follows any subsequent encounter with the organism.
  1. Instead of differentiating into antibody-producing plasma cells during the primary response, some B-cells persist as *memory cells*. These cells retain specificity for that particular antigen and produce a faster and larger version of the primary response during secondary antigen exposure.
  2. The generation of memory B-cells takes place in *germinal centers*.
  3. During the secondary response, a much larger amount of *IgG* is produced, and these levels persist much longer than during the primary response.

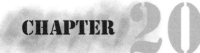

CHAPTER 20

Immunology: Clinical Concepts

I. HARMFUL IMMUNITY

The normal ability of the immune system to defend against infection relies on both the recognition and memory of a wide range of antigens, as well as strong, nonspecific mechanisms to mobilize and eliminate microbes. In certain situations, these important natural functions can act against the host, resulting in the following immunopathological reactions (Fig. 20-1).

A. Autoimmunity: Autoantibodies and Rheumatoid Disorders

Autoimmunity refers to the *loss of tolerance to self*. Many of these diseases stimulate self-reactive B-cells, giving rise to specific autoantibodies that may be detected clinically and help assist with diagnosis and management (Table 20-1).

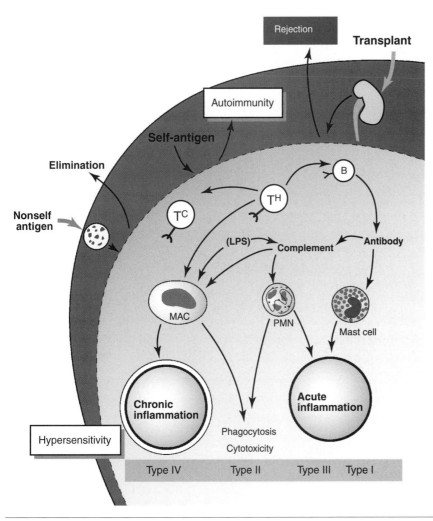

Figure 20–1 An overview of harmful immunity.

TABLE 20-1	Autoimmunity: Autoantibodies, and Rheumatoid Disorders		
DISEASES	AUTOANTIBODIES	CHARACTERISTICS	HARDCORE IMMUNOLOGY
Rheumatoid Arthritis	Rheumatoid factor (anti-IgG antibody) ANA	Symmetric inflammatory arthritis, worse in morning; primarily affects knee and hand MCP and PIP joints	RF = IgM anti-IgG, but is not specific for RA; titer does not correlate with disease activity
Systemic lupus erythematosus	ANA anti-ds DNA and anti-Smith (both highly specific for SLE)	Malar rash, photosensitivity, discoid rash, oral ulcers, arthritis, serositis, cerebritis, and glomerulonephritis	ANA > 98% sensitive; ANA is used for screening person suspected of having SLE; antiribosomal-P and antineuronal antibodies correlate to ↑ risk of lupus cerebritis; antiphospholipid antibodies can cause false-positive test in SLE and syphilis, and a falsely elevated PTT
Diffuse scleroderma	Anti-Scl-70	Diffuse fibrosis of the skin in the trunk and proximal extremities, and fibrosis of internal organs	Flexion contractures, ung/cardiac/renal fibrosis
Limited scleroderma (CREST syndrome)	Anti-centromere	**C**alcinosis **R**aynaud's phenomenon **E**sophageal motility disorder **S**clerodactyly **T**elangiectasias	Anti-centromere antibody is highly specific for limited scleroderma
Polymyositis/ dermato-myositis	Anti-Jo-1	Bilateral proximal muscle weakness; characteristic cutaneous manifestations (Grotton`s papules, heliotrope rash)	Increase risk of malignancy, especially in adult; dermatomyositis; inflammatory myopathy directed against capillaries (antibody-complement—mediated injury)
Sjögren`s syndrome	Anti-Ro Anti-La	Triad: Keratoconjunctivitis sicca (dry eyes), xerostomia (dry mouth), and arthritis	Immune-mediated destruction of salivary glands and lacrimal glands; thyroid-associated autoimmunity is common; associated with HLA-DR3
Wegener's granulomatosis	C-ANCA	Perforation of nasal septum, chronic sinusitis, otitis media, hemoptysis	Characterized by necrotizing granulomas in the lungs and upper airways and necrotizing glomerulonephritis; fatal if not treated
Polyarteritis nodosa	P-ANCA	Vasculitis of the small- to medium-size vessels that mainly affects the kidney	Associated with hepatitis B infection
Goodpasture disease	Anti-glomerular basement membrane (anti-GBM) antibody	Pulmonary-renal syndrome	Linear staining of glomerular basement membrane and alveolar basement membrane
Drug-induced lupus	Antihistone antibodies	Drugs implicated: procainamide, methyldopa, hydralazine, and isoniazid	Four cardinal features separate it from SLE: 1. Sex ratio is nearly equal 2. Nephritis and CNS involvement are not usually present 3. Low serum complement levels and antibodies against native DNA do not occur 4. Symptoms resolve when the offending drug is withdrawn

*PTT is falsely elevated in SLE because the lupus anticoagulant antibody binds to phospholipid that initi-ates clotting in the test tube.

Note: antinuclear antibodies; ANCA, antineutrophil cytoplasmatic antibody; CREST, calcinosis cutis, Raynaud's phenomenon, esophageal motility disorder, sclerodatyly, and telangiectasia; SLE, systemic lupus erythematosus.

B. Hypersensitivity

Hypersensitivity refers to an excessive immune response that leads to tissue or organ damage.

- **Type I—Acute hypersensitivity** (*allergic, anaphylaxis, immediate*)
  - Type I requires *two exposures* to the same specific antigen/allergen.
    1. The first exposure results in sensitization and the production of circulating IgE anti-bodies, which bind to receptors on mast cells and/or basophils.

2. Second exposure to the allergen results in *allergen-IgE complex on the surface of mast cells and/or basophils*, resulting in their degranulation and release of basophilic granules containing histamine and other vasoactive amines. This ultimately results in an immediate local (*allergic*) or systemic reaction (*anaphylaxis*).

○ Type I examples:

- Systemic anaphylaxis
- Allergic rhinitis and asthma
- Atopic dermatitis
- Penicillin allergy
- Food allergies (e.g., peanuts, shellfish)
- Local wheal and flare

- **Type II—Cytotoxic hypersensitivity (antibody dependent)**

○ During an immune response, antibodies formed are able to *recognize and attack the host's molecular component of cell surfaces and tissues* in one of two ways:

1. Direct recognition of a molecule on the host cell surface that is exposed secondary to injury, but is normally not visible to the immune system and thus becomes immunogenic.

2. An extrinsic nonantigen is absorbed onto the host's cell surface. When the immune system attacks the antigen on the cell surface, it leads to destruction of the antigen as well as the tissue the antigen is bound to.

○ Mediation occurs *via IgG or IgM bound with Ag on tissues*, resulting in the activation of the classical pathway complement deposition, and the production of multiple inflammatory mediators at this site.

○ The end result is cell death and lysis that occurs from the production of membrane attack complexes and phagocytosis following opsonization of the host tissue surface.

○ Type II examples:

- Autoimmune hemolytic anemia
- Drug-induced hemolytic anemia (e.g., methyldopa)
- Erythroblastosis fetalis—Rh-negative mother gives birth to an Rh-positive newborn. In subsequent pregnancies, IgG antibodies can cross the placenta and destroy fetal cells
- Transfusion reactions
- Myasthenia gravis
- Goodpasture's disease
- Graves' disease
- Hyperacute transplant reaction

- **Type III—Immune-complex hypersensitivity**

○ Occurs with an excess of antigens, which over time combine with antibodies to form soluble immune complexes.

○ When the amount of soluble immune complexes (Ag-Ab) in circulation increases to the degree that they become insoluble, *immune complexes begin to deposit in tissues, triggering complement activation*.

○ Activated complement, with Ag-Ab complexes, results in the neutrophilic degranulation of enzymes and *stimulation of macrophages* to release cytokines, reactive oxygen intermediates, and nitric oxide, leading to cell destruction and tissue damage.

○ Type III examples:

- Serum sickness
- Systemic lupus erythematosus (SLE) nephritis or vasculitis
- Immune complex glomerulonephritis
- Arthus reaction

- **Type IV—Cell-mediated hypersensitivity** (*delayed type*)

○ This is a *hapten-mediated reaction* that requires sensitization. After antigen reexposure, an APC (typically a macrophage) takes up the antigen and processes it on an MHC-I or MHC-II molecule, while also releasing IL-12, which promotes proliferation of T-helper cells.

○ A sensitized memory T-cell, either CD4+ Th1 (intracellular antigen) or CD8+ cytotoxic T-cell (extracellular antigen), initiates the reaction:

- Activation of a *sensitized Th1* cell releases *IFN g*, which leads to macrophage activation and further Th1 activation; and *IL-2*, which enhances T-cell proliferation.
- Activation of *sensitized cytotoxic T-cells* causes the direct destruction of target cells (*allograft rejection*).

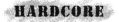

Labeling type II as antibody dependent is a misnomer, because types I to III are all antibody dependent.

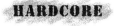

Type III reactions may also cause the activation of both the coagulation factor XII, resulting in coagulation and thrombosis; and the activation of kinin, causing vasodilation and edema.

TABLE 20-2	Common Associations of HLA with Immunodisease
DISEASE	**HLA ALLELE**
Hashimoto's disease	DR11
Graves' disease	DR17
Insulin-dependent diabetes	DQ8, DQ2/8, DQ6
Addison's disease	DR17
Rheumatoid arthritis	DR4
Juvenile rheumatoid arthritis	DR8
Ankylosing spondylitis	B27
Reiter's syndrome	B27
Myasthenia gravis	B8

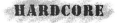

Individuals with thymic aplasia (DiGeorge syndrome) can have no sensitization.

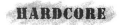

Type IV reaction will be apparent within 48 to 72 hours.

- The end result is a *cell-mediated immune response led by macrophages*.
  - Activated macrophages show increased phagocytic, bacteriocidal, and cytocidal activity.
  - If the reaction is due to chronic intracellular organism infections, the DTH response may be prolonged, resulting in the macrophages transforming into epithelioid and multinucleated giant cells, which is characteristic of a *granulomatous reaction*.
- Type IV examples:
  - Granulomatous diseases—Tuberculosis, sarcoidosis, leprosy
  - Purified protein derivative test (PPD)—Mantoux test/TB skin tests
  - Graft versus host disease (GVHD)
  - Contact dermatitis—Poison ivy, eczematous reaction
  - Organ allograft transplant rejection

C. Transplant Rejection

The normal role of T-cells to detect alterations in MHC antigens can lead to a recipient-mediated immune response against the transplanted tissue. Depending on the tissue, graft rejection may be mediated by either T- and/or B-cells, along with nonspecific effector molecules and cells including complement, cytotoxic cells, and macrophages. Successful organ transplant depends on matching donor and recipient MHC antigens as closely as possible and then suppressing the recipient's immune response.

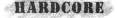

HLA-A and B antigens are used to predict the likelihood of long-term graft survival.

HARDCORE

Graft vascular disease involves the rapid development of graft arteriosclerosis from fibroblast proliferation, leading to intimal thickening and lumen stenosis.

- Types of transplant rejection can be divided into the following:
  - **Hyperacute rejection (immediate)**—Due to ABO mismatch or *pre-existing HLA antibodies* in the transplant recipient.
    - Occurs *within minutes* after transplant.
    - Pre-existing antibodies attach to and damage endothelial cells of the donor organ, causing vascular occlusion.
  - **Acute rejection**—An immune-mediated response. This cell-mediated reaction is due to *cytotoxic T-cells reacting against foreign MHCs*.
    - Occurs *weeks* after transplant.
  - **Chronic rejection**—A resulting vascular damage caused by antibodies. This type of rejection is *irreversible*.
    - Occurs *months to years* after transplant.
  - **GVHD**—If competent T-cells from the donor are transferred to an HLA-incompatible recipient, the grafted T-cells may recognize and attack host antigens.
    - Patients with GVHD develop rash, jaundice, diarrhea, severe oral-mucosal ulceration and scarring, and hepatosplenomegaly.

II. IMMUNODEFICIENCIES

Immunodeficiency disorders are more commonly encountered as secondary disease from drugs, malnutrition, or infections, but may also be caused by genetic disorders. Primary immunodeficiency disorders are categorized based on the type of immunologic cell that is deficient (Fig. 20-2).

A. Defects Involving Multiple Types of Cells

- **Ataxia telangectasia**—Deficiency of *T-cells and IgA* secondary to a deficiency of DNA repair.
  - Causes defects in the brain and skin.

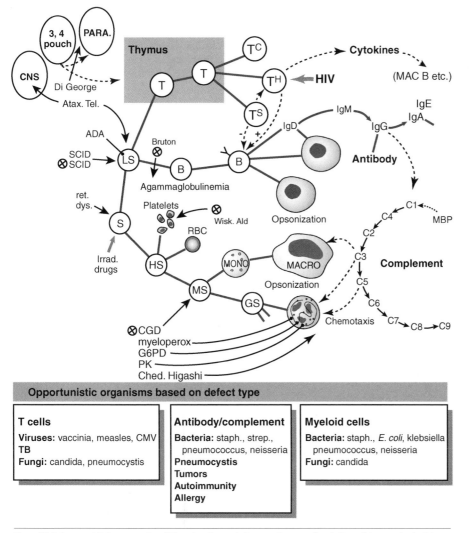

Figure 20–2 Immunodeficiency overview. Different patterns of disease arise according to the cell type predominately affected. Defects that affect several types of cells include reticular dysgenesis (ret. dys), SCID, ataxia telangiectasia (Atax Tel.), and Wiskott-Aldrich (Wisk. Ald). Defects predominately affecting B-cells include agammaglobulinemia and autoimmunity. Defects affecting T-cells include DiGeorge syndrome, purine nucleoside phosphorylase (PNP), and several cytokine defects. Defects affecting myeloid cells include chronic granulomatous disease (CGD), myeloperoxidase, glucose-6-phosphate dehydrogenase (G6PD), pyruvate kinase (PK), and Chediak-Higashi syndrome (Ched Higashi). In addition, defects can affect complement, including low levels of mannose-binding protein (MBP). Lymphoid stem cell (LS), hematopoietic stem cell (HS), stem cell (S), myeloid stem cell (MS), granulocyte stem cell (GS).

- ○ Common presentation is in a child between the ages of 5 and 10 years with spider veins on the skin, who acts "clumsy" and has an IgA deficiency.
- **Reticular dysgenesis**—Total failure of stem cells.
  - ○ These patients die soon after birth.
- **Severe combined immunodeficiency (SCID)**—Both T-cells and B-cells are defective. Some cases are X-linked, while others result from deficiency of adenosine deaminase (autosomal recessive) or the failure to synthesize MHC class II antigens or IL-2 receptors.
  - ○ Patients present with recurrent viral, bacterial, fungal, or protozoal infections.
- **Wiskott-Aldrich syndrome**—Characterized by a defect in a protein that regulates cytoskeleton function, resulting in *B- and T-cell deficiencies*.
  - ○ These patients develop eczema, platelet deficiencies, and deficient antibody response to capsular polysaccharides.

B. Defects Affecting T-Cells

- **Cytokine defects**—Principally caused by defects in cytokine receptors, these include IL-2 and IL-12 cytokines that limit the response of Th1 cells. These defects are very rare.

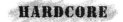

Some patients with SCID will be missing HLA class I or II from lymphocytes.

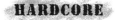

Wiskott-Aldrich serology will show elevated IgA, normal IgE, and low IgM.

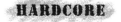

Wiskott-Aldrich patients are at a heightened risk of developing non-Hodgkins lymphoma.

- **DiGeorge syndrome**—Absence of thymus (*thymic aplasia*) and parathyroid glands from the failure of the third and fourth pharyngeal pouches to develop.
  - Patients present with symptoms of hypocalcemia (tetany) from absent parathyroid glands, or recurrent viral, fungal, or protozoal infections from lack of T-cells, as well as other facial, esophageal, and cardiac malformations.
- **Purine nucleoside phosphorylase (PNP) deficiency**—PNP is a salvage enzyme in T-cells, and when deficient, this allows nucleosides to accumulate and damage the cell.

C. Defects Affecting B-cells

- **Bruton's and variable agammaglobulinemia**—Bruton's type is characterized by the *total absence of B-cells*, while the variable type is caused by B-cell inability to *differentiate into plasma cells or to make one class of immunoglobulins* (most frequently IgA; germinal centers may be absent).
  - Bruton's is an *X-linked disease*, characterized by *recurrent pyogenic bacterial infections* (otitis media, sinusitis, pneumonia from *H. influenzae* and *S. pneumoniae*) in infancy.
  - Remember: **B**ruton's is a **B**-cell disorder in **B**oys (X-linked).
- **Hyper IgM immunodeficiency**—Results from the inability to convert IgM-producing B-cells to IgA, IgG, IgE-producing B-cells.
  - Serology will demonstrate highly elevated IgM, with low levels of all other antibodies.
- **IgG subclass deficiency**—Low levels of IgG result in recurrent otitis media, bacterial meningitis, and chronic lung infections. IgA deficiency is the most common subclass deficiency and can lead to sinus and lung infections.

D. Defects Affecting Myeloid Cells

- **Chediak-Higashi syndrome**—Polymorphs contain large granules but are *not able to properly form phagolysosomes*. May also have an impaired response to chemotaxis.
  - Autosomal-recessive disease that results in recurrent pyogenic infections by *streptococci and staphylococci species*. Infection can trigger an accelerating phase of unremitting T-cell proliferation that may require bone marrow transplantation.
- **Chronic granulomatous disease (CGD)—X-linked defect** of the oxygen breakdown pathway involving a cytochrome and lack of *NADPH oxidase activity*, resulting in neutrophil phagocyte deficiency.
  - Characterized by chronic infections with bacteria that *do not produce peroxide* (catalase +), including *S. aureus* and *E. coli*; also fungi.
- **Job's syndrome**—Results from *poor neutrophil chemotaxis*.
  - Patients present with *recurrent staphylococcal abscesses*.
- **Myeloperoxidase, glucose-6-phosphate dehydrogenase (G6PD), pyruvate kinase (PK)**—Genetic deficiencies in these enzymes result in recurrent infections with bacteria and fungi.

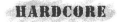

E. Complement Deficiencies (Table 20-3)

TABLE 20-3	Complement Deficiencies	
COMPLEMENT DEFICIENCY	**CLINICAL CORRELATES**	**HARDCORE IMMUNOLOGY**
C1 esterase	Hereditary angioedema	Overactive complement causes elevated esterase production
C1, C2, C4	Predispose to immune complex disease, particularly systemic lupus erythematosus	ANA is used for screening person suspected of having SLE
C3	Recurrent pyogenic sinus and respiratory tract infections	These patients are more susceptible to infection from encapsulated bacteria, including an elevated risk of developing sepsis from pyogenic *S. aureus*
C5–C8	*Neisseria* bacteremia	Not as severe as MAC deficiency
C5–C9 (MAC)	*Neisseria* sepsis	May be fatal
Mannose-binding protein	Severe childhood infections	MBP stimulates the classical cascade pathway and acts as an opsonin for phagocytosis
Decay activating factor, CD59	Paroxysmal nocturnal hemoglobinuria (PNH)	May present with "brown" urine following complement-mediated hemolysis

III. VACCINES AND VACCINATION

A. Types of Immunity

- **Passive immunity**—A *short-lived immunity* to infection provided by host acquisition of preformed antibodies from another individual, a different species, or from genetically engineered antibodies.
  - Advantage:
    - The humoral response is *immediate*.
  - Disadvantages:
    - The immunity against that specific antigen is lost quickly.
    - Memory is not established.
    - Potential to transmit infectious agents from donor serum.
  - Examples:
    - *Maternal antibody transfer*. Antibodies transferred from mother to infant via placental and infant intestinal absorption provide *protection for approximately the first 6 months of life*. Placental antibodies transferred are IgG. Intestinal antibodies transferred are IgA.
    - Pooled human antibody injections. Collection of human IgGs from various human plasma donors. Used as prophylaxis for patients with long-standing humoral immunodeficiency.
    - Antiserum against tetanus, hepatitis B, rabies, many snake bites.
- **Active immunity (vaccination)**—A long-lasting immunity to infection that follows the exposure to harmless forms of a microorganism. This results in the *development of memory cells* capable of expanding and providing protection if the microorganism is reencountered.
  - Advantages:
    - Immunity against the specific antigen is long-lasting.
    - Memory cells are produced.
    - Once immunity is established, subsequent response against the invading pathogen is rapid.
  - Disadvantage:
    - The immunity takes time to develop.
  - Examples:
    - Many types of vaccines (see below).

B. Types of Vaccines

- **Killed organisms**
  - Provides active immunity by *injecting killed, inactivated bacteria or viruses*.
  - Antigenicity of the organisms must be maintained during inactivation process.
  - Examples:
    - Killed Polio Vaccine (Sal**k vaccine**)
    - Cholera
- **Live attenuated organisms**
  - Mediated by a process in which an organism is modified so as to render it incapable of establishing an infection, but still capable of "*revving-up*" the immune system.
  - Replication of the organism inside the host results in a larger "dose" of the vaccine and thus a stronger immune response.
  - Examples:
    - Live polio oral vaccine (Sabin vaccine)
    - Measles-mumps-rubella (MMR)
- **Subunit vaccines**
  - Microorganisms contain *multiple antigenic molecules*. Subunit vaccines exploit one or few of these microorganism molecules, resulting in *active immunity*.
  - Examples:
    - Tetanus-diphtheria toxoid (TdT) vaccine
    - Acellular pertussis vaccine
    - Influenza subunit vaccine
    - Pneumococcal capsular subunit vaccine
    - Hepatitis A and B surface antigen vaccine

HARDCORE

Live vaccines are not recommended in immunodeficient individuals because they can result in full-blown disease.

- **Adjuvants**
  - Adjuvants are substances capable of *nonspecifically boosting the immune response to an antigen*. Adjuvants are injected simultaneously with antigen/vaccines to provide the immune system with a *slow-release depot of antigen*, activating the innate immune system and increasing antigen presentation.
  - Examples:
    - Aluminum salt compounds
    - Liposomes
    - Oil emulsions

Practice Questions and Answers

QUESTIONS

1. A 43-year-old immigrant presents to your clinic with facial edema, lymphadenopathy, and chest pain. You are concerned about the patient and admit him to the hospital. Soon after, the patient develops abdominal pain and is diagnosed with megacolon. You suspect that this patient may have Chagas' disease. Which vector is responsible for transmitting *Trypanosoma cruzi* to humans?
   A. Tsetse fly
   B. Mosquito
   C. Black fly
   D. Reduviid bug
   E. *Chrysops* fly
   F. Sandfly

2. A 27-year-old female arrives in the emergency room complaining of severe lower abdominal pain. She describes the pain as sharp, midgastric, and radiating towards her groin. The pain is the most severe when she is ambulating, requiring her to shuffle from foot-to-foot when walking. She also reports fever up to 38.5°C during the past few days, and has nausea but no vomiting. After some questioning, the patient states that she has had moderate vaginal discharge for the past few weeks, and has a history of sexually transmitted diseases. Physical exam reveals a yellow vaginal discharge with a strong odor. Her cervix appears red and raw, and she is exceptionally tender during manual movement of her cervix. No visible lesions are present. Cultures of the vaginal discharge are taken. Which of the following descriptions is the most consistent with this infecting organism?
   A. Naked, icosahedral double-stranded circular DNA virus
   B. Lactose-fermenting gram-negative bacilli
   C. Pear-shaped flagellated protozoa
   D. Intracellular obligate intracellular parasite
   E. Spirochetes on dark-field microscopy

3. A 5-year-old boy presents to your clinic with a draining wound on the planter aspect of his right foot. The wound is round, erythematous, and draining a small amount of purulent discharge. On further questioning, the patient reports stepping on a nail that pierced his tennis shoe one week earlier while playing on his school playground. All of his vaccinations are up to date. Which of the following organisms is most likely infecting this patient's foot wound?
   A. *Staphylococcus aureus*
   B. *Streptococcus epidermitis*
   C. *Cornybacterium*
   D. *Pseudomonas aeruginosa*
   E. *Candida albicans*
   F. *Eikenella corrodens*

4. An elderly woman develops a urinary tract infection. She delays treatment and soon becomes hypotensive, tachycardic, and nonarousable. She is quickly brought into the emergency room where she is diagnosed with gram-negative septic shock. Which component of the *E. coli* bacterium is responsible for increasing the host formation of cytokines, leading to bacteremia and septic shock?
   A. Capsule
   B. ST toxin
   C. LT toxin
   D. Fimbria
   E. Lipopolysaccharide

5. While rotating on the HIV service you see a 32-year-old patient with acquired immunodeficiency syndrome who has been closely followed in the clinic for the past 4 months. The patient is complaining of severe, nonresolving diarrhea for the past week. You obtain a stool sample and see acid-fast oocysts that are not gray or greasy. What is the most likely causative organism?
   A. Enterohemorrhagic *Escherichia coli*
   B. *Salmonella*
   C. *Giardia*
   D. Enterotoxic *E. coli*
   E. *Cryptosporidium*
   F. *Cryptococcus*

6. Two patients arrive in the emergency room complaining of vomiting and watery diarrhea for the past 3 hours. The patients report that they consumed breaded chicken and fried rice from a street vendor at a Chinese New Year celebration about 5 hours before the onset of the symptoms. Which of the following is the most likely causative agent?
   A. *Staphylococcus aureus*
   B. *Giardia lambia*
   C. *Salmonella enteritidis*
   D. Norwalk agent
   E. *Shigella*
   F. *Bacillus cereus*

7. When culturing a sputum sample from a 67-year-old patient in the intensive care unit, the laboratory finds that the sample stains blue with Gram stain. Further analysis indicates that this sample is a catalase-negative coccus, which causes partial (alpha) hemolysis to red blood cells (RBCs). Which of the following organisms is most likely the organism causing infection?
   A. *Staphylococcus aureus*
   B. *Staphylococcus epidermidis*
   C. *Streptococcus pyogenes*
   D. *Streptococcus pneumoniae*
   E. *Peptostreptococcus*
   F. *Pseudomonas aeruginosa*
   G. *Bordetella pertussis*

8. A 28-year-old law student presents to your clinic complaining of 6 weeks of intermittent, intense epigastric pain. The patient states that the pain initially began while he was preparing for midterm exams. On further questioning, you discover that the pain is worse before meals or a few hours after meals. You suspect that the patient may be suffering from a duodenal ulcer. Which of the following enzymes enables the possible causative organism to colonize the human gastrointestinal tract?
   A. Urease
   B. Lipase
   C. Hemolysins
   D. Hyaluronidase
   E. Staphylokinase

9. An elderly woman who is in the intensive care unit for urosepsis develops 2 days of massive diarrhea. She has been on several antibiotics since she was admitted to the hospital, and you suspect that she may have developed a colonic infection of *Clostridium difficile*. *C. difficile* produces two toxins, toxins A and B. Which of the following actions do these toxins have?
   A. Toxin A inhibits translation of human mRNA and toxin B increases cAMP.
   B. Toxin A hemolyzes RBCs and Toxin B inhibits acetylcholine release.
   C. Toxin A increases fluid secretion and inflammation and toxin B is cytotoxic to colonic epithelial cells.
   D. Toxin A increases cGMP, inhibiting resorption of NaCl, and toxin B binds GM1 gangliosides on intestinal cell membranes.
   E. Toxin A ribosylates elongation-factor (EF-2), and toxin B activates membrane G-proteins, activating adenylate cyclase.

10. A 32-year-old woman comes to your clinic complaining of burning with urination and an increasing frequency of urination. A Gram stain of her urine is performed, which isolates an organism that is gram-positive. Which of the following is the most likely organism that is causing this urinary tract infection?
   A. *Staphylococcus aureus*
   B. *Staphylococcus saprophyticus*
   C. *Streptococcus pyogenes*
   D. *Enterococcus faecalis*
   E. *Proteus mirabilis*

11. Investigative laboratory techniques have isolated an enveloped DNA virus, with a large, dumb-bell-shaped genome that replicates in cytoplasm. Which of the following is the most likely virus isolated by this laboratory?
    A. *Retroviridae*
    B. *Orthomyxoviridae*
    C. *Parvoviridae*
    D. *Poxviridae*
    E. *Papovaviridae*

12. A 12-year-old boy presents to the emergency room with a fever, severe headache, and confusion. When obtaining a history from his parents, you discover that these symptoms began the day before, after the patient went swimming with friends in a freshwater pond. The patient is admitted to the hospital, but rapidly deteriorates and a lumbar puncture is performed. Subsequent cerebrospinal fluid analysis reveals "slug-like" amoebas. Which of the following is the most likely organism infecting this patient?
    A. *Acanthamoeba*
    B. *Naegleria fowleri*
    C. *Leishmania donovani*
    D. *Toxoplasma gondii*
    E. *Giardia lambia*

13. While working at a women's clinic for immigrants, a young women unexpectedly delivers a jaundiced infant who is found to have hepatosplenomegaly, thrombocytopenic purpura, pneumonitis, and CNS damage. Which of the following congenital infections does this neonate most likely have?
    A. *Toxoplasma gondii*
    B. *Treponema pallidum*
    C. *Rubivirus*
    D. Cytomegalovirus
    E. Herpes simplex virus

14. A 42-year-old alcoholic presents to the emergency room complaining of chest pain, fever, chills, cough, and myalgia. The patient reports that her cough has been producing rust-colored, mucoid sputum. Her temperature in the ER is 40°C and she has an elevated white blood cell count, which is predominantly neutrophils. An alpha-hemolytic, lancet-shaped, gram-positive diplococcus is isolated on blood agar. Which of the following is the most likely causative agent?
    A. *Legionella pneumophila*
    B. *Streptococcus pneumoniae*
    C. *Neisseria meningitidis*
    D. *Mycoplasma pneumoniae*
    E. *Klebsiella pneumoniae*

15. After hiking through a national park in the southeastern United States, a 26-year-old male develops a fever, sore throat, headache, nausea, and a rash on the lower parts of both his arms and legs. When he arrives to the emergency room, he is febrile and complaining of wrist and ankle swelling along with his initial rash. Which of the following is this patient most likely suffering from?
    A. Streptococcal pharyngitis
    B. Epidemic typhus
    C. Lyme disease
    D. Q fever
    E. Rocky Mountain spotted fever

16. An 11-year-old boy presents to your clinic complaining of a fever, rash, and conjunctivitis for the past 5 days. Physical examination reveals a sickly looking boy with a maculopapular rash over his abdomen and lower back. His mother reports that the rash was originally located over his neck and thorax, but seems to have moved distally. In addition, you notice small bluish spots on the buccal mucosa. Which virus family is responsible for these symptoms?
    A. *Bunyaviridae*
    B. *Orthomyxoviridae*
    C. *Paramyxoviridae*
    D. *Rhabdoviridae*
    E. *Caliciviridae*
    F. *Togaviridae*

17. A 43-year-old burn victim develops fever, chills, and an elevated white blood cell count. On physical examination, the patient is found to be tachycardic, but his lungs sound clear and he has strong and equal pulses. Cultures of his blood, wounds, and urine are sent to the laboratory. The blood and urine cultures do not grow any organisms, but the wound cultures grow a non-lactose fermenting, gram-negative rod. Which of the following is the most likely organism cultured?
    A. *Proteus mirabilis*
    B. *Klebsiella pnemoniae*
    C. *Pseudomonas aeruginosa*
    D. *Escherichia coli*
    E. *Serratia marcescens*

18. While working for the state center of disease control, you are asked to give a presentation about disease transmission and prevention of various zoonotic organisms. During your presentation, what do you portray as the most appropriate and effective way for reducing the transmission of toxoplasmosis?
    A. Avoid intravenous drug abuse
    B. Avoid swimming in contaminated water
    C. Avoid using human excrement as vegetable fertilizer
    D. Cook fish and seafood thoroughly
    E. Heat all canned foods to 60°C
    F. Avoid cat litter or take proper care in changing litter

19. While working in the surgical intensive care unit, you are closely monitoring a 43-year-old patient who has sustained a splenic laceration, partial small bowel transaction, and a closed head injury 6 days earlier after a roll-over motor vehicle collision. Early during her hospital stay, she began a regimen of clindamycin for an intraabdominal abscess that grew *B. fragilis* on culture. About 4 days later, the patient developed severe, foul-smelling diarrhea. Another culture is sent and the patient is found to have a *Clostridium difficile* infection. How does *C. difficile* cause diarrhea?
    A. *C. difficile* invades the colonic mucosa, surviving intracellularily and causing disease in a mechanism similar to that of *Listeria*.
    B. *C. difficile* invades the colonic mucosa and secretes two surface toxins inside the colon.
    C. *C. difficile* stacks itself on the colonic surface to cause maladsorption and the appearance of a pseudomembrane.
    D. *C. difficile* exotoxins damage the cells, causing a disruption in transport and attracting polymorphonuclear cells to cause the appearance of a pseudomembrane.

20. A 62-year-old patient with a history of rheumatic fever as a child undergoes extensive oral surgery, but does not take the perioperative prophylactic antibiotics he was prescribed. Two weeks later, the patient develops low-grade fever, tachycardia, a new systolic murmur and several episodes of syncope. Which of the following is the most likely causative agent?
    A. *Enterococcus faecalis*
    B. *Staphylococcus aureus*
    C. *Streptococcus viridans*
    D. *Streptococcus agalactiae*
    E. *Streptococcus pneumoniae*
    F. *Streptococcus pyogenes*

21. A 2-year-old boy arrives at your clinic with a serious otitis media infection. After speaking with his parents, you learn that this is his fifth otitis media infection and that the boy also has a history of boils and has been hospitalized twice with pneumonia. Cultures isolate *H. influenzae* and serum analysis reveals that this boy has an absence of all five immunoglobulin classes. Which of the following hereditary immune deficiency diseases do you diagnose this patient with?
    A. Neutropenia
    B. AIDS
    C. Chronic granulomatous disease
    D. Bruton's X-linked agammagobulinemia
    E. Severe combined immunodeficiency disease

22. A 9-year-old boy presents to his pediatrician with fatigue, easy bruising, and bony pain at night. He is subsequently diagnosed with leukemia and undergoes a bone-marrow transplant. The boy receives bone marrow stem cells from his HLA-matched sister, but develops a syndrome characterized by pancytopenia, aplastic anemia, skin rash, oral ulcers, diarrhea, and jaundice. What did this boy develop?
    A. Graft-versus-host disease
    B. Hyperacute rejection

C. Acute rejection

D. Failure of bone marrow engraftment

E. Secondary infection

23. A 43-year-old male presents to the emergency room following an altercation in which he was hit in the arm with a wrench, resulting in a 3-inch laceration but no fracture. After cleaning and suturing the laceration, you question the patient regarding his tetanus vaccination status. He reports that he received the tetanus immunization 7 years ago and was given a tetanus booster 4 months ago after cutting himself with a broken bottle. What treatment should be administered to this patient at this time?

A. Tetanus toxoid and human antitoxin should be administered.

B. Tetanus toxoid should be administered.

C. Human toxin should be administered.

D. Horse toxoid should be administered.

E. Nothing should be administered to this patient.

24. Which of the following immunoglobulin (Ig) classes is the first to be produced in an immune response to an antigen?

A. IgA

B. IgG

C. IgM

D. IgD

E. IgE

25. Which of the following fragments are seen when immunoglobulin G (IgG) is cleaved by papain?

A. Two monovalent fragments with antibody activity—antigen-binding fragments (Fab)

B. Two fragments devoid of antibody activity

C. Fab fragments that contain the variable (V) section of the heavy chain but not the light chain

D. Fab fragments that contain the variable (V) section of the light chain but not the heavy chain

E. Two crystallizable fragments (Fc) and one Fab fragment

ANSWERS

1. D

The reduviid bug spreads *Trypanosoma cruzi* to humans, which can result in the development of Chagas' disease, classically characterized by facial swelling, lymphadenopathy, myocarditis, and megacolon. The tsetse fly (answer A) is the vector for *Trypanosoma rhodesiense* and *gambiense*, which causes sleeping sickness. Mosquitoes (answer B) are vectors for a multitude of infectious organisms. The black fly (answer C) is the vector for *Onchocerca volvulus*, which causes river blindness. The *Chrysops* fly (answer E) is the vector for *Loa loa*, which causes loiasis. The sandfly (answer F) is the vector for *Leishmania*, which causes leishmanisis.

2. D

This is the classic presentation of pelvic inflammatory disease (PID), which is most commonly caused by *Chlamydia trachomatis* and *Neissiera gonorrhoea*. The description provided in the question is that of *C. trachomatis*. *C. trachomatis* is an ATP-defective organism that survives intracellularly. Diagnosis is made by visualizing cytoplasmic inclusions on Giemsa stain. Answer A refers to human *Papillomavirus*, which is the most common STD in the United States, but does not cause vaginal discharge. Answer B refers to *E. coli*, which also does not cause PID. Answer C is consistent with *Trichomonas vaginalis*, a protozoan parasite that causes watery vaginal discharge, but would also be expected to result in erythema of the external vagina but not the cervix. Answer E refers to *Treponema pallidum*, which produces a rash and chancre depending on the stage of infection.

3. D

Pseudomonas aeruginosa infection is classically associated with the type of injury described in this question stem: skin puncture by a rusty nail through a tennis shoe. Although the other organisms listed as answer choices are normal skin flora, *P. aeruginosa* is the most likely infecting organism with this type of injury.

4. E

Lipopolysaccharide molecules are located in the bacterial outer membrane of gram-negative rods and are responsible for increasing the bacterium resistance to the bacteriacidal activity of complement. Lipopolysaccharide also stimulates host macrophages to produce cytokines, particularly IL-1 and TNF, which are responsible for causing host fever, shock, and sepsis. The bacterial capsule (answer A) is responsible for neonatal meningitis; the ST and LT toxins (answers B and C) act on enterocytes to stimulate fluid secretion, resulting in diarrhea; and the fimbria (answer D) assist the bacteria in colonization.

5. E

Acid-fast oocysts are seen in infections with the protozoan *Cryptosporidium*, which causes severe, nonresolving diarrhea in patients with acquired immunodeficiency syndrome. It is also the most common cause of diarrhea in AIDS patients.

6. F

Vomiting and watery diarrhea can be caused by *B. cereus*, which is classically encountered after eating fried rice. Onset of vomiting and diarrhea occur within 6 hours after consumption of infected rice and is caused by a preformed heat-stable enterotoxin. *S. aureus* (answer A) causes symptoms within 4 to 6 hours of ingestion, and is typically associated with egg salad, cream pastries, and coffee creamers. *G. lambia* (answer B) causes foul-smelling and fatty diarrhea (steatorrhea) from drinking infected stream water. *Salmonella* (answer C) causes bloody diarrhea following the ingestion of eggs and poultry. Norwalk agent (answer D) causes vomiting from shellfish and contaminated prepared foods. Shigella (answer E) causes bloody diarrhea via fecal–oral contamination.

7. D

S. pneumoniae is a gram-positive coccus that grows in chains, is catalase-negative, and is alpha-hemolytic. *S. aureus* and *S. epidermidis* (answers A and B) grow in clusters and are catalase-positive. *S. pyogenes* (answer C) is catalase-negative but beta-hemolytic. *Peptostreptococcus* (answer E) does not cause hemolysis. *Bordetella pertussis* and *P. aeruginosa* (answers E and F) are gram-negative, and thus Gram stain pink.

8. A

The *H. pylori* organism is a common cause of duodenal ulcers. This organism produces urease, which neutralizes stomach acid and enables the organism to colonize the GI tract. This is also why a urease breath test is used to identify the presence of *H. pylori*. *H. pylori* does not contain any of the other enzymes listed as answer choices.

9. C

C. difficile contains two toxins: toxin A, which increases fluid secretion and inflammation; and toxin B, which is cytotoxic to colonic epithelial cells. Diptheria toxin inhibits the translation of human mRNA (answer A). *Vibrio cholegan* and *E. coli* heat-stable toxin increase cAMP levels (answer A). Hemolysins hemolyze RBCs, botulinium toxin inhibits acetylcholine release (answer B). *E. coli* heat-stable toxin and staphylococcal heat-stable toxin both increase cGMP and inhibit the resorption of NaCl (answer D). *E. coli* heat-stable and cholergen toxin bind GM1 ganglio-sides on intestinal cell membranes (answer D). Diptheria toxin ribosylates elongation-factor (EF-2), and pertussis toxin, which activates membrane G-proteins, activates adenylate cyclase (answer E).

10. B

S. saprophyticus is a gram-positive coccus that causes urinary tract infections in sexually active young women, and is the second most common cause of UTI and cystitis in this population after *E. coli*.

11. D

Poxviridae is a DNA virus that is enveloped, has a dumbbell-shaped genome, and replicates in the cytoplasm. This family includes the smallpox virus and molluscum contagiosum virus. *Retroviridae* and *Orthomyxoviridae* (answers A and B) are both RNA viruses. *Parvoviridiae* (answer C) and *Papovaviridae* (answer E) are both naked DNA viruses.

12. B

Naegleria fowleri is an amoeba that causes primary meningoencephalitis (PAM). This occurs most commonly in children who are diving or swimming in fresh water during hot weather. Patients develop fever, severe headaches, and confusion and can rapidly deteriorate, resulting in coma and death in a few days. CSF analysis reveals "slug-like" amoebas. *Acanthamoeba* (answer A) is also an amoeba, but is acquired from contact lens saline and causes ocular pain. *Leishmania* (answer C) is a blood protozoan spread by sandflies. *Toxoplasma gondii* (answer D) is a protozoan spread by ingestion of undercooked meat or cat feces, and *Giardia lamblia* (answer E) is a protozoan that is acquired in untreated water and results in diarrhea with malabsorption.

13. D

CMV can cause a generalized infection of infants resulting in neonatal jaundice, hepatosplenomegaly, thrombocytopenia purpura, pneumonitis, and CNS damage. *T. gondii* (answer A) results in congenital chorioretinitis, hydrocephalus, and intracranial calcifications. *T. pallidum* (answer B) causes neonatal syphilis characterized by fetal stillbirth, hydrops fetalis, frontal bossing, short maxilla, high palatal arch, or the Hutchinson triad: Hutchinson teeth (blunted upper incisors), interstitial keratitis, and eighth-nerve deafness. *Rubivirus* (answer C) is the causative agent of rubella and congenital *Rubivirus* infection that may result in neonatal deafness, cataracts, patent ductus arteriosus, neurologic sequelae, or thrombocytopenia. Congenital herpes simplex virus (answer E) can result in hypotension, jaundice, DIC, apnea, and shock.

14. B

S. pneumoniae is a lancet-shaped, gram-positive diplococcus that is alpha-hemolytic and a common cause of gram-positive pneumonia in substance abusers.

15. E

Rocky Mountain spotted fever is caused by *Rickettsia rickettsii* and is characterized by a rash that begins on the hands and feet of infected individuals. The other infectious diseases listed are not associated with a rash on the hands and feet.

16. C

The infectious disease described is measles. Measles causes an acute generalized disease char-acterized by a maculopapular rash that migrates cranially to caudally, fever, respiratory distress, and Koplik's spots on the buccal mucosa. Measles is a member of the *Paramyxoviridae* family. *Bunyaviridae* (answer A) contains the California encephalitis virus, the La Crosse encephalitis virus, and the *Hantavirus*. The *Orthomyxoviridae* (answer B) family contains the influenza viruses. The *Rhabdoviridae* (answer D) family contains the rabies virus. The *Caliciviridae* (answer E) family contains the Norwalk virus. *Togaviridae* (answer F) contains *Rubivirius* and *Alphavirus*.

17. C

Pseudomonas aeruginosa is a non-lactose fermenting, gram-negative rod that, as an opportunistic pathogen, commonly colonizes burn patients. The other answer choices are also gram-negative rods, but all are lactose-fermenting.

18. F
Toxoplasmosis is spread through both contaminated cat litter (pregnant women) and the ingestion of undercooked meat (immunocompromised people).

19. D
C. *difficile* causes the production of exotoxins, which result in diarrhea and the formation of a pseudomembrane. These infections commonly follow a regimen of antibiotics, particularly clindamycin, because these medications deplete the normal colonic flora and allow for colonization of C. *difficile*.

20. C
Streptococcus viridans is a normal component of the human oral flora. In patients with previously damaged heart valves, such as from rheumatic fever, S. *viridans* can attach to the injured valve after gaining access to the bloodstream (e.g., following dental work), resulting in subacute endocarditis.

21. D
Patients affected with Bruton's X-linked agammagobulinemia are unable to synthesize immunoglobulins of any isotype and suffer from recurrent pyogenic infections beginning at the age of 6 to 8 months when maternal antibody levels decline. The defect occurs in the tyrosine kinase enzyme. These patients do not have surface Ig-bearing B-cells in the peripheral blood and no plasma cells in lymph nodes. Patients with neutropenia (answer A) and AIDS (answer B) do not have a decrease in immunoglobulin levels. Patients with chronic granulomatous disease (answer C) have neutrophil phagocyte deficiencies but normal Ig levels. Patients with severe combined immunodeficiency (answer E) will be defective in both T-cells and B-cells resulting from a deficiency of adenosine deaminase (autosomal-recessive) or the failure to synthesize MHC class II antigens or IL-2 receptors.

22. A
Graft-versus-host disease follows the transfer of immunocompetent T-cells into an immunologically immature or incompetent recipient. Cytopenia, rash, diarrhea, and oral ulcers are characteristic of this condition. Hyperacute rejection (answer B) occurs within minutes after transplant and results in vascular occlusion. Acute rejection (answer C) occurs weeks after transplant and is characterized by an attack against donor tissue. Failure of bone marrow engraftment (answer D) or secondary infection (answer E) would not result in this clinical picture.

23. E
This patient has recently received a booster and currently has plenty of antitoxin in his blood; therefore he does not need any tetanus prophylaxis. If this patient had not received a tetanus booster in the last 5 years, he would need one at this visit.

24. C
IgM is the first antibody class to be produced in response to an antigen, and is the predominant antibody in the primary immune response. This response is followed by the production of either IgG or IgA during the secondary immune response.

25. A
Papain splits IgG to produce two antigen-binding fragments (Fab) and a crystallizable fragment (Fc). Because the Fab is monovalent, antigen can be bound by the Fab but not cross-linked and precipitated. A Fab fragment contains the variable (V) region of both the heavy and light chains.

APPENDIX A

Antimicrobial Pharmacology

This appendix provides a brief outline of antimicrobial agents commonly used within the world of medical microbiology. Understanding antimicrobial pharmacology is undoubtedly vital for peak performance both on the USMLE Step 1 examination and in clinical practice. Although an in-depth review of antimicrobial agents is outside the scope of this book, please see the *Hardcore Pharmacology* text for an effective and fast review of antimicrobial pharmacology.

I. ANTIBIOTICS

A. Cell Wall Synthesis Inhibitors (Table A-1)

These compounds block the final step in bacterial cell wall synthesis by binding to and inhibiting *transpeptidase enzymes*, which are responsible for cross-linking of the peptidoglycan subunits of the bacterial cell wall. Inhibition of the transpeptidase enzyme is the common mechanism of action for all cell wall synthesis inhibitors, except for *vancomycin*. Additionally, these compounds also activate bacterial enzymes called *endogenous autolysins* that are normally involved in the degradation and remodeling of the bacterial cell wall. Because transpeptidases are also inhibited, enzymatic degradation of the cell wall by autolysins continues without reconstruction. All of the cell wall inhibitors are considered *bactericidal*.

- Natural penicillins—*penicillin G, penicillin G benzanthine, penicillin G procaine, penicillin V*
- β-lactamase-resistant penicillins—*methicillin, nafcillin, oxacillin, dicloxacillin, cloxacillin*
- Extended-coverage penicillins—*amoxicillin, ampicillin*
- Anti-pseudomonal penicillins—*carbenicillin, ticarcillin, piperacillin*
- β-lactamase inhibitors—*clavulanic acid, sulbactam, tazobactam*
- Penicillin combined with a β-lactamase inhibitor—*ampicillin/sulbactam, amoxicillin/clavulanic acid, piperacillin/tazobactam*
- Carbapenems—*imipenem, meropenem, ertapenem*
- Monobactam—*aztreonam*
- Vancomycin
- Cephalosporins—*first, second, third, fourth generations*

B. Protein Synthesis Inhibitors (Table A-2)

The continual production of proteins is essential for growth and survival of all cells. Bacterial production of proteins is dependent on a *70S ribosome* (humans have an 80S particle) to translate mRNA into polypetides. This 70S ribosome consists of two subunits: a *large 50S* and a *small 30S* subunit. Protein synthesis inhibitors target either of these subunits. All protein synthesis inhibitors (except the aminoglycosides) are considered *bacteriostatic*.

- Macrolides—*erythromycin, clarithromycin, azythromycin*
- Aminoglycosides—*gentamicin, trobamycin, amikacin, streptomycin, spectinomycin*
- Tetracyclines—*tetracycline, doxycycline, minocycline, demeclocycline*
- Chloramphenicol
- Streptogramins
- Oxazolidiones—*linezolid*

TABLE A-1   Cell Wall Synthesis Inhibitors

DRUG CLASS	DRUGS	HARDCORE BUG TARGETS	MECHANISM OF ACTION	MAJOR SIDE EFFECTS
Natural Penicillins	*Penicillin G* *Penicillin V*	• Gram (+) cocci/rods • Gram (−) cocci • Spirochetes	Inhibition of transpeptidases	Anaphylaxis, erythema multiforme, hemolytic anemia
β-Lactamase-Resistant Penicillins	*Methicillin* *Nafcillin* *Oxacillin* *Dicloxacillin* *Cloxacillin*	• Gram (+) cocci	Inhibition of transpeptidases	Liver toxicity, thrombophlebitis, interstitial nephritis
Extended-Coverage Penicillins	*Amoxicillin* *Ampicillin*	• Gram (+) cocci/rods • Gram (−) cocci • Spirochetes • Greater activity against gram (−) bacilli	Inhibition of transpeptidases	Rashes and diarrhea
Anti-pseudomonal penicillins	*Carbenicillin* *Ticarcillin* *Piperacillin*	• Gram (−) rods • Anaerobes	Inhibition of transpeptidases	Hypokalemic alkalosis, platelet dysfunction
Penicillin Combined with a β-Lactamase Inhibitor	*Ampicillin/sulbactam Amoxicillin/clavulanic acid, Piperacillin/ tazobactam*	• Gram (+)	Inhibition of transpeptidases	Same as above for each specific constituent of the combination; β-lactamase inhibitors are not associated with significant side effects
Carbapenems	*Imipenem-cilastin* *Meropenem* *Ertapenem*	• Broad spectrum • Aerobes • Gram (+) • Gram (−) • Anaerobes	Inhibition of transpeptidases	Imipenem is nephrotoxic if not given with cilastin, seizures
Monobactams	*Aztreonam*	• Aerobic gram (−) rods	Inhibition of transpeptidases	Pain at injection site, thrombocytopenia
Vancomycin	*Vancomycin*	• Aerobic gram (+) • Anaerobic gram (+)	Inhibition of peptidoglycan synthesis	Thrombophlebitis, neutropenia, red man syndrome
Cephalosporins			Inhibition of transpeptidases	Allergic reactions/rash and pseudomembranous colitis
1st generation	*Cefazolin* *Cephalexin*	• High gram (+), limited gram (−)		
2nd generation	*Cefuroxime* *Cefoxitin* *Cefotetan*	• Decreased gram (+), increased gram (−)		Disulfuram like reaction with cefotetan
3rd generation	*Ceftriaxone* *Cefotaxime* *Ceftazidime*	• Increasingly limited gram (+) • Increased gram (−)		Cholelithiasis with ceftriaxone
4th generation	*Cefepime*	• Increased gram (+), increased gram (−)		

TABLE A-2   Protein Synthesis Inhibitors

DRUG CLASS	DRUGS	HARDCORE BUG TARGETS	MECHANISM OF ACTION	MAJOR SIDE EFFECTS
Macrolides	*Erythromycin* *Azythromycin* *Clarithromycin*	• Gram (+) • Atypicals • Minimal gram (−)	Inhibition of **50S** ribosomal subunit	Diarrhea, prolongation of the QT interval → torsades de pointes, erythromycin strongly inhibits CYP-450
Aminoglycosides	*Gentamicin* *Tobramycin* *Amikacin* *Streptomycin* *Spectinomycin*	• Gram (−) • Enteric bacteria *Pseudomonas*	Inhibition of **30S** ribosomal subunit	Ototoxicity (irreversible), nephrotoxicity
Tetracyclines	*Tetracycline* *Doxycylne* *Minocycline* *Demeclocycline*	• Broad spectrum • Gram (+) • Gram (−) • Anaerobes, atypical bacteria, protozoa, parasites	Inhibition of both **30S** and **50S** ribosomal subunits	Photosensitivity, decreased bone growth, teeth discoloration
Clindamycin	*Clindamycin*	• Aerobic gram (+) cocci • Anaerobes	Inhibition of **50S** ribosomal subunit	Severe diarrhea, pseudomembranous colitis
Chloramphenicol	*Chloramphenicol*	• Broad spectrum	Inhibition of **50S** ribosomal subunit	Dose-related bone marrow suppression, aplastic anemia, gray baby syndrome
Streptogramins	*Quinupristin-dalfopristin*	• Gram (+) • Atypicals • Minimal gram (−)	Inhibition of **50S** ribosomal subunit	Pain and erythema at injection site, liver enzyme elevation, prolongation of QT interval
Oxazolidinones	*Linezolid*	• Gram (+) • Anaerobes	Inhibition of **70S** ribosomal initiation-complex	Reversible thrombocytopenia, serotonin-like syndrome

TABLE A-3	DNA Synthesis Inhibitors			
DRUG CLASS	**DRUGS**	**HARDCORE BUG TARGETS**	**MECHANISM OF ACTION**	**MAJOR SIDE EFFECTS**
Fluoroquinolones			Inhibition of topoisomerase II (DNA gyrase) and topoisomerase IV	Photosensitivity, QT prolongation → torsades de pointes, impaired cartilage development (*therefore not to be used during pregnancy or for children*)
2nd generation	*Norfloxacin Ofloxacin Ciprofloxacin*	• Gram (–) • Gram (+) • Genitourinary		
3rd generation	*Levofloxacin Gatifloxacin Moxifloxacin*	• Gram (–) • Gram (+) genitourinary • Respiratory bugs • Typicals		
4th generation	*Trovafloxacin*	• Gram (–) • Gram (+) • Respiratory • Genitourinary • Atypicals • Anaerobes		Fatal liver toxicity
Sulfonamides	*Trimethoprim-sulfamethoxazole (TMP-SMX) Sulfadiazine Sulfisoxazole*	• Enteric gram (–) • Limited gram (+)	*Trimethoprim*: inhibition of dihydrofolate reductase *Sulfa drugs*: inhibition of dihydropteroate synthetase	Photosensitivity, Stevens-Johnson syndrome, hemolytic anemia in patients with G6PD deficiency, leukopenia

C. DNA Synthesis Inhibitors (Table A-3)

Obviously, these agents act to inhibit bacterial DNA synthesis. The quinolones (first generation) and fluoroquinolones (second through fourth generations) prevent DNA synthesis by inhibiting **topoisomerase type II** (also known as DNA gyrase) and **topoisomerase type IV**, and are active against gram-negative bacteria and intestinal pathogens, but also possess increasing activity against gram-positive and atypical bacteria from the first to the fourth generations. Fourth-generation *fluoroquinolones* are also active against anaerobes and are considered a broad-spectrum antibiotic. Sulfonamides inhibit **dihydropteroate synthetase**, the enzyme responsible for the conversion of PABA to folic acid, while trimethoprim inhibits **dihydrofolate reductase**, the enzyme responsible for the conversion of dihydrofolate to tetrahydrofolate (*trimethoprim-sulfamethoxazol, TMP-SMX, is administered as one synergistic agent*).

- Quinolones (first generation) and fluoroquinolones (second through fourth generations)
    - First generation—*nalidixic acid (not used clinically or tested on Step 1)*
    - Second generation—*norfloxacin, ofloxacin, ciprofloxacin*
    - Third generation—*levofloxacin, gatifloxacin, moxifloxacin*
    - Fourth generation—*trovafloxacin*
- Sulfonamides—*trimethoprim-sulfamethoxazole(TMP-SMX), sulfadiazine, sulfisoxazole*
- *Nitrofurantoin*

II. ANTIFUNGALS

Antifungals (Table A-4) target both fungi rigid cell walls, containing **chitin and glucan** and cell membranes, which contain **ergosterol** (a derivative of cholesterol). These agents may be administered systemically or topically.

TABLE A-4	Antifungals			
DRUG CLASS	**DRUGS**	**HARDCORE BUG TARGETS**	**MECHANISM OF ACTION**	**MAJOR SIDE EFFECTS**
Subcutaneous and Systemic Antifungals	*Amphotericin B*	• *Candida* • *Cryptococcus* • *Histoplasmosis* • *Blastomyces* • *Coccidioides* • *Aspergillus*	Binds fungal cell ergosterol-forming membrane pores, fungicidal	Nephrotoxicity, hypotension, anemia, thrombophlebitis
	Capsofungin	• *Aspergillus* • *Candida*	Inhibition of β-1,3 glucan synthase	Pruritis bronchospasm

(Continued)

TABLE A-4	Antifungals (cont.)			
DRUG CLASS	**DRUGS**	**HARDCORE BUG TARGETS**	**MECHANISM OF ACTION**	**MAJOR SIDE EFFECTS**
Flucytosine	• Chromomycoses	Pyrimidine antimetabolite, • *Candida* • *Cryptococcus* • *Aspergillus*	Neutropenia, thrombocytopenia converted to 5-FdUMP that inhibits thymidylate synthase and the production of DNA, fungicidal	due to bone marrow suppression
	Terbinafine	• Onychomycoses • Dermatophytes	Blocks ergosterol synthesis by inhibiting squalene epoxidase, fungicidal	Loss of taste
Superficial Antifungals	Nystatin	• *Candidiasis*	Binds to ergosterol, disrupts fungal membranes altering permeability and leading to cell lysis	Rare topically
	Griseofulvin	• Dermatophyte infections • Tinea capitis	Inhibits fungal microtubule function	Pancytopenia
	Naftifine	• Dermatophyte • Onychomycoses	Inhibits squalene epoxidase/fungal sterol biosynthesis	Neutropenia, lymphopenia
Imidazoles—General and Topical	Clotrimazole Miconazole Ketoconazole	• *Candida* • *Cryptococcus* • Histoplasmosis • *Blastomyces* • *Coccidioides* • Dermatophytes	Inhibits fungal cytochrome P450, fungicidal	Local irritation
Systemic Imidazoles	Fluconazole	• *Coccidiodes*	Inhibits fungal cytochrome P450, fungicidal	Stevens-Johnson syndrome
	Itraconazole	• *Aspergillus*		Idiosyncratic hepatitis
	Ketoconazole	• *Candida*		Gynecomastia, hepatic toxicity
	Voriconazole	• *Aspergillus*		Blurred vision, photophobia, altered color perception

- Subcutaneous and systemic antifungals—*amphotericin B, capsofungin flucytosine capsofungin, terbinafine*
- Topical antifungals—*nystatin, griseofulvin*
- Imidazoles
  - Systemic imidazoles—*fluconazole, itraconazole, ketoconazole, voriconazole*
  - Topical imidazoles—*clotrimazole, miconazole, ketoconazole*

III. ANTI-MYCOBACTERIALS

Remember that the mycobacteria are rod-shaped, aerobic bacteria that cause tuberculosis, leprosy, and infections common in immunocompromised patients. The treatment of active tuberculosis is a commonly tested concept and consists of a four-drug regimen designed to prevent drug resistance (Table A-5).

- Drugs for TB—*rifampin, isoniazid, pyrazinamide, ethambutol/streptomycin* (RIPE/S)
- Drugs for leprosy—*dapsone, clofazimin*

TABLE A-5	Anti-Mycobacterials			
DRUG CLASS	**DRUGS**	**HARDCORE BUG TARGETS**	**MECHANISM OF ACTION**	**MAJOR SIDE EFFECTS**
Antituberculosis	Rifampin	• *M. tuberculosis* • *M. leprae* • *Nisseria* • *H. influenzae* type B	Inhibits bacterial RNA by binding mycobacterial DNA-dependent RNA polymerase, bacteriocidal	Hepatotoxicity, bodily secretion discoloration
	Isoniazid	• *M. tuberculosis* • *M. bovis* • *M. kansasii*	Inhibits the synthesis of mycolic acid, bacteriocidal	Hepatotoxicity, peripheral neuropathy
	Pyrazinamide	• *M. tuberculosis*	Inhibits fatty acid synthetase I (FASI) of *M. tuberculosis*, bacteriocidal	Hyperuricemia, body secretion discoloration
	Ethambutol	• *M. tuberculosis* • *M. avium-intracellulare* • *M. bovis* • *M. kansaii*	Inhibits cell wall arabinogalactan, bacteriostatic	Color blindness

(Continued)

TABLE A-5	Anti-Mycobacterials (cont.)			
DRUG CLASS	**DRUGS**	**HARDCORE BUG TARGETS**	**MECHANISM OF ACTION**	**MAJOR SIDE EFFECTS**
	Streptomycin	• *M. tuberculosis* • Gram (–) enterics *Pseudomonas* • *Francisella tularemis* • *Yerstinia Pestis Brucella abortis*	Binds the **30S** subunit of the bacterial ribosome	Ototoxicity, nephrotoxicity
Antileprosy	*Dapsone*	• *M. leprae*	Inhibits bacteria folic acid synthesis	Methemoglobinemia, erythema multiforme
	Clofazimin	• *M. leprae* • *M. avium*-complex • *M. bovis* • *M. fortuitum*	Binds and inhibits mycobacterial DNA replication, enhances immuno phagocytosis	Bowel obstruction, skin discoloration

IV. ANTIVIRALS

Viruses are tiny infectious units that contain only one type of nucleic acid (RNA or DNA) and posses an envelope with a protein coat that forms a capsid. Although viruses are responsible for a vast number of different diseases, the pharmaceutical treatments available are relatively few (Tables A-6 and A-7).

- Drugs for respiratory viral infections—*amantadine, rimantadine, zanamivir, oseltamivir*
- Drugs for herpes infections—*acyclovir, valaciclovir, penciclovir, famciclovir, valganciclovir, ganciclovir, cidofovir, foscarnet, idoxuridine, trifluridine*

TABLE A-6	Antivirals: Respiratory, Anti-HSV/VZV, Anti-CMV, Ophthalmic Antiherpetics, Antihepatitis			
DRUG CLASS	**DRUGS**	**HARDCORE BUG TARGETS**	**MECHANISM OF ACTION**	**MAJOR SIDE EFFECTS**
Respiratory Antivirals	*Amantadine Rimantadine*	• Influenza A	Inhibits viral uncoating	Seizures, heart failure, orthostatic hypotension
	Zanamivir Oseltamivir	• Influenza A and B	Inhibits neuraminidase	Bronchospasm in asthmatics
	Ribavirin	• Respiratory syncytial virus (RSV) • Hepatitis C virus (HCV) • *Orthomyxoviridae* • *Paramyxoviridae* • *Arenaviridae*	A nucleoside analog that inhibits the replication of RNA viruses	Hemolytic anemia, dyspnea
• **Antiherpes Simplex Virus (HSV) 1 and 2** • **Anti-Varicella-Zoster Virus (VZV)**	*Acyclovir Valacyclovir Peniclovir Famciclovir*	• HSV • VZV • CMV prophylaxis for posttransplant patients with valacyclovir	Activated by thymidine kinase, ultimately inhibits viral DNA polymerase	Rarely encephalopathy with seizures
Anti-Cytomegalovirus (CMV)	*Ganciclovir Valganciclovir*	• CMV	Specific to thymidine kinase encoded by CMV, inhibits viral DNA polymerase	Bone marrow suppression, granulocytopenia, thrombocytopenia
	Foscarnet	• CMV • HSV • VZV	Acts as an inorganic pyrophosphate molecule inhibiting viral DNA and RNA polymerase	Nephrotoxicity
	Cidofovir	• CMV	Acts as a cytosine nucleotide analogue, leading to viral DNA chain termination	Nephrotoxicity
Ophthalmic Antiherpetics	*Idoxuridine*	• HSV	Incorporated into viral DNA leading to chain termination	Eye irritation
	Trifluridine	• HSV	Inhibits viral thymidylate synthase conversion of dUMP → dTMP, inhibiting viral DNA replication	Eye irritation
Antihepatitis	*Lamivudine*	• HIV • HBV	Inhibits reverse transcriptase (RT), causes chain termination by incorporating into the growing viral DNA	Rarely pancreatitis in children
	Adefovir	• HBV	Reverse transcriptase inhibitor, interferes with HBV viral RNA-dependent DNA polymerase	Hematuria
	Interferon alpha	• HBV • HCV • HDV	Inhibits viral replication, increases immuno-phagocytosis, increases cytotoxicity of lymphocytes	Flu-like symptoms, depression, bone marrow suppression

TABLE A-7	Antivirals: HIV			
DRUG CLASS	**DRUGS**	**HARDCORE BUG TARGETS**	**MECHANISM OF ACTION**	**MAJOR SIDE EFFECTS**
Nucleoside Reverse Transcriptase Inhibitors (NRTIs) the "-vudine" drugs	*Zidovudine (AZT) Tavudine Didanosine Lamivudine Abacavir Zalcitabine*	HIV	Inhibits reverse transcriptase, incorporated into growing the HIV DNA leading to chain termination	Lactic acidosis; **zidovudine:** anemia, neutropenia, hepatitis; **zalcitabine:** peripheral neuropathy, pancreatitis; **abacavir:** hypersensitivity reaction
Nucleotide Reverse Transcriptase Inhibitors (NtRTIs)	*Tenofovir*	HIV	Inhibits HIV reverse transcriptase	Muscular weakness
Non-Nucleoside Reverse Transcriptase Inhibitors (NNRTIs) the "-vir-" drugs	*Efavirenz Nevirapine Delavirdine*	HIV	Inhibits HIV reverse transcriptase by conformational change	Insomnia, hepatotoxicity
Protease Inhibitors the "-navir" drugs	*Saquinavir Ritonavir Indinavir Nelfinavir Amprenavir Lopinavir Atazanavir*	HIV	Inhibits HIV protease enzyme	Cushignoid-like appearance, hepatotoxicity, kidney stones
Viral Entry Inhibitors	*Enfurvitide*	HIV	Inhibits fusion of the HIV-1 virus with CD4 cells	Insomnia

- Drugs for hepatitis B and C infections—*lamivudine, adefovir, ribavirin, interferon alpha*
- Drugs for HIV infections:
  - Nucleoside reverse transcriptase inhibitors (NRTIs)—*zidovudine (AZT), tavudine, didanosine, lamivudine, abacavir, zalcitabine*
  - Nucleotide reverse transcriptase inhibitors (NtRTIs)—*tenofovir*
  - Non-nucleoside reverse transcriptase inhibitors (NNRTIs)—*efavirenz, nevirapine, delavirdine*
  - Protease inhibitors—*saquinavir, ritonavir, indinavir, nelfinavir, amprenavir, lopinavir, atazanavir*
  - Viral entry inhibitors—*enfurvitide*

V. ANTIPARASITICS

Parasitology encompasses a wide variety of infectious diseases and organisms, including protozoa, plasmodium, and worms (helminths) (Table A-8).

- Antimalarials—*primaquine, cholroquine, quinine, quinidine, mefloquine*
- Anticestodes—*niclosamide*
- Antiflagellates—*metronidazole, nifurtimox, suramin, pentavalent antimony*
- Antinematodes—*ivermectin, mebendazole, pyrantel pamoate, thiabendazole*
- Antitrematodes—*praziqantel*

TABLE A-8	**Antiparasitics**			
Drug Class	**Drugs**	**Hardcore Bug Targets**	**Mechanism of Action**	**Major Side Effects**
Antimalarials	**Primaquine**	• *Plasmodium* tissue schizonticide	Oxidizes reduced glutathione	Granulocytopenia
	Cholroquine	• *Plasmodium* blood schizonticide (erythrocytic malaria)	Inhibits RBC allowing the accumulation of soluble heme, also decreases parasitic DNA synthesis	Nightmares, nail bed discoloration
	Quinine Mefloquine	• *Plasmodium* blood schizonticide	Depresses parasitic oxygen/carbohydrate uptake and metabolism, disrupts parasitic replication and transcription	Cinchonism
	Proguanil Primethamine	• *Plasmodium* blood schizonticide	Folate antagonists that inhibit dihydrofolate reductase	Rash, GI distress, pruritis
Anticestodes	Niclosamide	• *D. latum* • *Taenia* species (tapeworm infections)	Inhibits parasitic anaerobic phosphorylation of ADP in mitochondria	
Antiflagellates	Metronidazole	• Giardia • Amoebic dysentery • *Gardnerella vaginalis* • *Trichomonas* • *Clostridium difficile*	Forms reduced cytotoxic compounds that bind and are toxic to parasitic proteins and DNA	Disulfiram reaction with alcohol
	Nifurtimox	• *T. cruzi*	Generates intracellular oxygen radicals	Anaphylaxis, neuropathy
	Suramin	• African trypanosomiasis (sleeping sickness)	Inhibits enzymes involved in parasitic energy metabolism	Renal toxicity
Antinematodes	Ivermectin	• Onchocera volvulus (river blindness)	Increasing parasitic GABA receptor activation	Hypotension, dizziness
	Mebendazole	• Whipworm • Hookworm • Pinworm • Roundworm	Interferes with parasitic synthesis of microtubules	Rare
	Pyrantel Pamoate	• Roundworm • Pinworm • Hookworm	Depolarizing neuromuscular nicotinic receptors	GI distress
	Thiabendazole	• *Trichinella* • *S. stercoralis* (threadworm)	Interferes with parasitic microtubular aggregation	Erythema multiforme, Stevens-Johnson syndrome
Antitrematodes	Praziqantel	• Trematodes	Increases permeability of the parasitic cell membrane to calcium causing paralysis	GI distress

Index

Page numbers followed by *f* refer to illustrations; page numbers followed by *t* refer to tables.